THE
HEALING ARTS

To the blessed memory of Lam Pui Yin, my godmother, and to
Phyliss Wydra and Ray Kunz-Lechner, my aunts.

Ted Kaptchuk

To the many practitioners of the Healing Arts who have used their
skills for me; starting with the doctor who hauled me feet first into
the world.

Michael Croucher

THE
HEALING ARTS

A Journey Through the Faces of Medicine

TED KAPTCHUK and MICHAEL CROUCHER

BRITISH BROADCASTING CORPORATION

Acknowledgements

We would like to thank the many healers around the world who shared their experience and knowledge with us. And we are grateful to the Lemuel Shattuck Hospital for making it possible for Ted to work with the BBC. We are also grateful to the following people for their help in preparing this book: Sheila Ableman, editor; Tamasin Day-Lewis and Michael York, film directors; Nancy Trichter, literary agent; Harvey Blume and Randy Showstack, critics; Beth Poisson, librarian, and last, but not least, Bob Burger for being a last-minute magician.

The objects in the cover photograph are all on display in the Wellcome Museum of the History of Medicine at the Science Museum in South Kensington. We acknowledge the co-operation extended by this Museum in providing these objects for photography.

Published by the British Broadcasting Corporation
35 Marylebone High Street, London W1M 4AA

ISBN 0 563 20355 2 (hardback)
ISBN 0 563 20447 8 (paperback)

First published 1986

© Ted Kaptchuk and Michael Croucher 1986

Set in 11 on 13pt Imprint by Phoenix Photosetting, Chatham
and printed in England by Mackays of Chatham

Colour originated and printed by Belmont Press, Northampton

CONTENTS

PREFACE

The skill of the physician lifteth up his head,
So that he standeth in the presence of princes.
God has created medicines out of the earth,
And let not a man of discernment despise them.
My son, in sickness be not negligent.
Pray unto God, for He can heal,
And also give a place to the physician.
And let him not be far from thee, for there is indeed need of him,
For there is a time when success is in his power.

Jeshua Ben-Sir, Ecclesiasticus, *Chapter 37 (c. 180 BC)*

The authors of this book came to their subject from quite different backgrounds and perspectives. Michael Croucher is British and has been a television producer for more than twenty years. In the course of producing a documentary for the BBC he met, and was treated by, doctors practising traditional forms of medicine in Japan, China and India. His long interest in medicine led him to attend a lecture in London in 1983, shortly after returning from the Far East. The speaker was a young American doctor who had established an unusual, multi-faceted clinic in a Boston hospital that is affiliated to several major medical schools. Ted Kaptchuk's medical certification is not, however, in the orthodox medicine of his country, but in oriental medicine. After undergraduate studies in the United States he pursued his own journey of discovery in the Portuguese colony of Macao in southeast China, not far from Hong Kong. He learned the language and was adopted into a Chinese family. Back in his own country, his mastery of herbalism and acupuncture placed him in demand in the enthusiasm for things Chinese during the 1970s.

After that lecture in 1983 Michael Croucher and Ted Kaptchuk discussed the possibility of bringing the full range of the world's medical perspectives to the attention of the public. The result is a television series, *The Healing Arts*; this book is an attempt to enlarge on those documentaries, offering the detail and scope that only a book can provide.

In spite of, or perhaps because of, their diverse backgrounds, the co-authors have arrived at a statement about medicine that is exciting in both its practical and theoretical implications. In brief, it is that each medicine that man has produced, including the scientific medicine of today, has a validity of its own and cannot be subsumed into any other. By its very nature, any medicine is only partial – a mirror of the people who created it, an expression of what they thought of themselves or believed about their world. The medicine of the scientific tradition is a powerful one, but it reflects our limitation to an analytical view of the world that ignores many other facets of life. This statement is a profoundly hopeful one. It represents a rejection of the tunnel vision that attempts to fit snatches of this or that form of medicine into whatever kind is currently dominant.

Apart from the last two and a half chapters of the book, 'I' on the following pages is Ted Kaptchuk, for the simple reason that he is the medically experienced half of the partnership and most of what is said in these pages relates to the practical experience of healing. But it is the hope of both authors that this book will help dispose of some of the encrusted prejudices and blinding assumptions that continue to burden the healing arts.

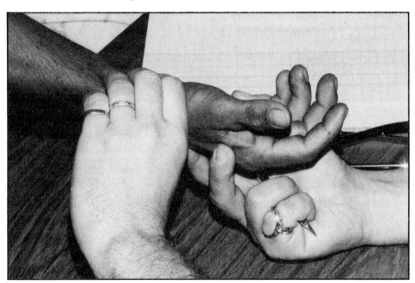

The study of a patient's pulse is central to diagnosis in Oriental traditional medicine and it is examined in great detail in their ancient texts

INTRODUCTION

A glance at the contents page of this book might lead the reader to think that it is no more than a discussion of the bizarre or unusual developments in health care, leading up to our own medical model, with a dash of Eastern medicine thrown in for spice. Let me dispel that idea straightaway.

I have been privileged to see the healing arts at work at many levels and from many perspectives: studying and practising in the Far East, lecturing and consulting throughout Europe, and working in the clinic I helped to found in the United States. As a result I have a profound belief in the merit and current applicability of every system of medicine in the world. More than thirty different therapies are used at my Pain and Stress Relief Clinic at the Lemuel Shattuck Hospital in Boston. These different faces of medicine have been assembled not only to enable a comparison to be made of their efficacy, but also for their synergistic effect and its benefits to the patients. It is our intention at the clinic that practitioners of each of the healing arts develop their viewpoint from the implicit challenge of the other systems.

The first distinction I want to make is between the idea of an inevitable progression of human thought and that of a simultaneous development on many fronts. Acceptance of the first idea leads to the dominance of a single system – in the developed countries, what I have called scientific medicine. The second of these concepts, and the one for which I will argue in this book, implies the existence of a multiplicity of systems of varying merit, but of great mutual value when taken together in their entireties.

Second, I must distinguish between two ways of delivering this multiplicity of healing arts. The commonly used word 'holistic' seems to refer to that approach which acknowledges the importance of the subjective element in medical treatment, and holistic practitioners often bring many therapies to bear on the health problems of their patients. In dealing with the whole person this medical

8

ideology has attracted millions of people who have felt modern medicine to be too fragmented. Our clinic, on the other hand, seeks to deal with such fragmentation by bringing practitioners together but allowing each of them to be distinct. While we recognise the inherent limitations of each approach, the mathematics of the best healing does not comprise the addition of the inner world of the patient to the objective data. Healing involves a special 'magic' of skill, timing, sensitivity and humility that each of the healing arts can embody. If a phrase is needed to characterise this approach, I would call it multi-dimensional, pluralistic or integrated medicine.

Third, I would like to make the distinction between illness and disease. By blurring the distinction we sometimes preclude some types of treatment, and even forget what healing is all about. In this book, I would like to maintain that illness is the state of a patient, beyond discomfort, but defined in the patient's terms. Disease is an objective condition, independent of the patient's judgement, which many medical models often assume to be the whole of illness.

Finally, because I am a doctor of oriental medicine there may be some confusion about the standpoint adopted by this book. Though it would be simple to depict it as yet another West discovers East odyssey, or even East rediscovers West, it would not be accurate. I believe that East and West are only two of the many intriguing pathways to be taken through the complexity of health and illness.

With regard to modern scientific medicine, I reiterate what I expressed in *Chinese Medicine: The Web That Has No Weaver*:

> Western science can be criticised for insensitivity, for arrogance, for storming Heaven – but the fact remains that it is humble, and humility is integral to the best scientific thought. For all its misuses, the idea of progress implies that not everything has been achieved, that more is yet to come. In order to remain science, science must believe that what it discovers tomorrow may undermine and revolutionise everything it believes today. Western science, unlike traditional Chinese thought, is necessarily receptive to the new.

I respect science and also actively participate in research, its most important ritual. Yet I am continually called to other, older forms of healing, some still at work, though disguised, in modern medicine, and most of them openly outside it. It is an error to try to reduce these medical traditions to a core of scientifically authenticated fact fleshed out by mistakes and superstition. Scientific validity is not necessarily more important than aspects of a tradition that science may find indifferent or antagonistic. The efficacy and beauty of each approach is revealed only when considered in its entirety.

Modern man has a long way to go in recognising other healing arts.

9

The fact that modern medicine borrows from its ancient and modern competitors does not, in my opinion, validate those alternatives. The relaxation response, for example, leans heavily on meditation techniques perfected in the East; but this does not mean that the scientific stamp has been put on meditation. Similarly, the major ingredient of modern decongestants, ephedrine, was reinstated in Western pharmacology in the 1920s after having been thrown out with the whole of herbalism centuries before; but the point is not that ancient herbalism can be shown to be scientific here and there.

This type of fragmentation is compounded by difficulties created by the dominance of one medical system. Any alternatives to the orthodoxy of the day are systematically excluded from general public testing and are under-represented in medical schools and are, for additional reasons, disparaged in practice. For a time in the 1970s the reopening of relations between the USA and China led to a resurgence of interest in such techniques as acupuncture, but even such well-researched areas of Western medicine as nutrition and massage are today considered quite secondary to drug therapy.

Our Boston clinic is far from being the only major institution to explore other areas of medicine. In the United Kingdom, so-called complementary medicine has several organisations working to broaden medical alternatives. One new group, the Research Council for Complementary Medicine, sees as its aim to position 'such long-standing and well-structured therapies as acupuncture, chiropractic, homeopathy, medical herbalism, naturopathy and osteopathy' not as alternatives to orthodox medicine but as therapies to work alongside it. In the United States, efforts to change the mainstream of medicine have been pioneered at the Brunswick Hospital in Amityville, New York, by Dr Joseph Beasley, author of the Ford Foundation publication *The Impact of Nutrition, Lifestyle and Environment on the Health of Americans*. Yet in these and other instances I see a distinct difference from our clinic's programme. I do not think it is just a fine point: I believe that the mainstream of medicine cannot be identified with any one medical system; rather, the mainstream is formed by all the tributaries. Is it even right to assume that there should be a mainstream at all? Perhaps we need to keep the natural rivers running freely, rather than dammed and confined.

A new perspective on the healing arts is needed, and a story concerned with the recent artificial heart transplants makes this point well. It is the epitome of technological accomplishment to construct a plastic heart to mimic the human organ. When the second recipient of such a transplant suffered a stroke, many explanations were given for the blood-clotting and subsequent paralysis. Later, the president of the American Stress Foundation offered a new point of view; in a letter to *The New York Times* he pointed out that the heart is more than just a mechanical pump. Among other things it produces a hormone, auriculin, that regulates fluid retention in the body. Lacking such regulation, fluid pressure on the arteries can precipitate blood-clotting and stroke. Pascal may have been more than poetical, the president added, when he said, 'The heart has its reasons, of which reason knows nothing.'

This book will explore many varieties of the healing arts. Since there are so many ways of approaching the phenomena of health and illness it is easy to find oneself in the same quandary to which physicists have grown so accustomed in this century. Is light made of particles? Is it made of energy? Are we body? mind? molecules? spirit? structure? behaviours? mind–body? Maybe when the famous mind–body split is overcome we will have as much trouble describing it as I now do in defining a multi-dimensional medicine.

In speaking of the contradictory healing models in modern psychiatry Leon Eisenberg, of Harvard Medical School, also alluded to modern physics:

> We lack the equivalent of Lorentz transformation equations that would enable us to move from one inertial frame of reference to another. A comprehensive and inclusive general theory of disease–illness . . . has yet to be written; even then it will be no more than a provisional guide for comprehending the clinical world.

It is even more true if one looks at the array of ideas and practices that comprise the healing arts. In the meantime, we have to open ourselves to different traditions in spite of, or rather because of, their dissimilarity to each other. We have to allow them to breathe. And we have to control our urge to rush them into premature synthesis.

The human body is more than a machine, and the human being is more than the sum of its bodily parts. An exploration of the healing arts must also involve the unknown – heavy-handed certainty excludes what can startle us and possibly even heal us. In the words of Werner Heisenberg, one of the founders of quantum physics, 'In the history of human thinking the most fruitful developments frequently take place at those points where two different lines of thought meet.' In every age, each medical pioneer thought he was the culmination of medical progress; what I hope to show here is that in the most hopeful sense each represents only a beginning.

1·THE· BALANCED·WAY

As I stood on the steps of the Arignar Anna Government Hospital of Indian Medicine in Madras, the meaning of a simple observation was forcefully brought home to me. Throughout China and India, medical students are required to study Western, scientific medicine along with their traditional systems. I had worked many years before in Chinese hospitals and had just come from another visit to some of India's teeming wards. I had seen the nearby medical complexes of Westerners. I knew that there was an 'English hospital' elsewhere in Madras. But here before me was a sprawling range of buildings – in-patient wards, out-patient clinics, herbal pharmacies, scientific research facilities, administrative offices – that physically confronted me with the seriousness, the urgency, the complexity of Eastern healing arts. This was no dying tradition, yet what medical school in Britain or the United States would ask its students even to acknowledge its existence?

I had worked in Ayurvedic hospitals before, and now I had come to visit one of the largest of them in India's fourth largest city. This morning, as on every morning, hundreds of people were standing in tightly compressed lines waiting for a consultation; they had chosen one of three Indian medical systems: Ayurvedic, Siddha or Unani. Inside, the crowds became even more suffocating. Still, I sensed intensity and dedication in the medical staff to whom I was introduced, a warm cohesiveness that is often missing in medical centres where each patient has the privacy, and the distancing, of personal attention.

I was offered the opportunity of accompanying Dr P. K. Rethidevi, in charge of Ayurvedic medicine here, on her rounds. A woman of forty-five, wearing a traditional sari, she immediately put me at my ease with her eagerness to share her experience and knowledge. She realised that Ayurvedic, literally the 'knowledge of longevity', is not as familiar to Westerners as are the acupuncture and

12

herbalism of Chinese medicine. Indeed, I explained that on a recent visit to a Chinese hospital my host had himself been surprised by my interest in Ayurvedic, which was not known to him. Unfortunately Westerners often view the Far East as a geographical, racial and intellectual entity; even the expression 'Far East' is a Western euphemism that serves to evade the diversity of southeast Asia.

Dr Rethidevi's first patient was a sixty-three-year-old former policeman who had had a stroke a month before; he was accompanied by an anxious daughter. When his family had first found him, lying in a coma on the floor by his bed, he had been rushed to the nearby Western hospital. There he had recovered consciousness, but his left arm and leg were paralysed and his speech was slightly impaired. Physiotherapy had helped, but on the advice of one of the Western doctors his family had decided to try Ayurvedic, in particular its famous medicated massage and oil baths.

I saw a man of angular build with a dry, rough complexion. His intense, penetrating, dark eyes made me feel that he had been a firm rather than a gentle keeper of the peace. Dr Rethidevi noted his flushed face and his thinness. She found his left side still inflexible, but his right side quite strong. He could speak only with difficulty, but even those poorly formed words revealed a determination to overcome his impairment. Though he complained of headaches, dizziness and constipation, he still had an excellent appetite.

After a few more questions Dr Rethidevi asked the nurse to show her a urine sample from that morning; it was dark yellow and concentrated. With a dropper she added a speck of sesame oil, which spread on the surface in concentric rings. 'This confirms my suspicion of fire and wind,' she told me, knowing that I was familiar with these concepts. If the oil had formed pearl-like droplets, she explained, the condition would be 'phlegm and watery' and would have indicated another range of treatment, usually more complex.

At last she took his pulse, which she described as active, jumpy and 'fast, like a frog'. She invited my diagnosis. 'In China,' I said, 'I would have called it wiry, like a taut violin string.' We enjoyed comparing the metaphors of the two cultures.

The fire and wind diagnosis – *pitta* and *vata* accordingly – were her symbols of observation. The former are heat and dehydration qualities, the latter movement qualities; in this patient they were out of balance. Because of a long-term fire disharmony, she said, the wind qualities of the body had suffered and in turn blocked bodily 'channels of energy', hence the stroke. Basically, the patient was too hot.

13

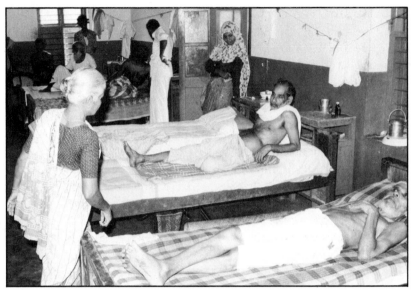

Dr Rethidevi on her rounds in the Arignar Anna Government Hospital, Madras

Without further elaboration, the doctor prescribed four herbal preparations, each compounded of several ingredients. One of the herbal formulas, designed to 'cool the fire', was first noted in a ninth-century Indian manual. The preparations prescribed to 'harmonise the wind' were recorded in a classic medical work whose origins were lost several centuries before Christ. The last and major prescription was panchakarma, a month-long physical therapy session of quite a different kind.

Each morning for an hour and a half the panchakarma, which is basically a sort of sauna treatment, proceeded; variations were introduced along the way. The ex-policeman, wearing only a loincloth, lay on a bed-size, screened box resembling nothing so much as a large barbecue pit; beneath him herbs smouldered and steam rose. Covered by a blanket, the patient began to sweat profusely. He was then removed to a '*dhroni* bed', a solid wooden pallet carved to fit the human body. Here he was treated to an unusual form of massage and anointing. Using small sachets of grain soaked in herbal oils, a man on each side gently pummelled the patient from head to toe. A wick dropped other liquids on to his forehead from a clay basin suspended over his head. The overwhelming impression was that the entire body was being caressed and nurtured.

I was irresistibly reminded of a classic account of a very different encounter between East and West. This time it was in the West, at the Yale Medical Center in New Haven, Connecticut. The author was the celebrated surgeon-poet Richard Selzer. 'On the bulletin board in the front hall of the hospital where I work,' he wrote, 'there appeared an announcement. "Yeshi Dhonden", it read, "will make the rounds at six o'clock on the morning of June 10".' Yeshi Dhonden was the personal physician of the Dalai Lama.

Tibetan medicine derives from a conference in the seventh century AD, history's first attempt at medical unification. Indian, Chinese and Persian-Greek doctors presented their methods, and the Tibetans grafted them on to their indigenous magical methods. Yeshi Dhonden's urine analysis is Greek in origin, his pulse-taking Chinese and his theories Indian, while his concentration-purification comes from the shaman and Buddhist world.

Of the 'whitecoats' who showed up, Selzer wrote, most had an air of 'ill-concealed dubiety and suspicion of bamboozlement'. But the doctor duly appeared, 'a short, golden, barrelly man dressed in a sleeveless robe of saffron and maroon'. For the past two hours Yeshi Dhonden had bathed, fasted and prayed to purify himself for his task, which was to examine a patient taken at random and explain his diagnosis to the hospital staff afterwards.

After introductions and a request for a urine sample, the visiting doctor moved to the bedside and entered into a trance-like vigil over the woman. At last this visual 'examination' gave way to the taking of her pulse. Selzer wrote:

> His eyes are closed as he feels for the pulse. In a moment he has found the spot, and for the next half hour he remains thus, suspended above the patient like some exotic golden bird with folded wings, holding the pulse of the woman beneath his fingers, cradling her hand in his. All the power of the man seems to be drawn down into this one purpose. . . . And I know that I, who have palpated a hundred thousand pulses, have not felt a single one.

A small wooden bowl and two sticks were produced, and a small specimen of the urine poured into the bowl; Yeshi Dhonden then whisked it like a sushi sauce until he made it foam. He smelt it three times before turning to leave. The woman, straining to rise from her bed, called out, 'Thank you, doctor', touching with her other hand the place where he had taken her pulse. No other words were spoken.

In the conference room immediately afterwards, the moment of truth had come. What was the diagnosis? Through a translator, the explanations sounded monk-like, furtive, poetic. Winds had been coursing through the body of the woman, currents breaking against barriers, eddying. They were in the blood, and were the signs of an imperfect heart. Long before she was born, Yeshi Dhonden explained, 'a wind had come, had blown open a deep gate that must never be opened. Through it charge the full waters of her river.' A lecturer then asked for the formal diagnosis of the hospital staff. 'Congenital heart disease,' he was told. 'Intraventricular septal defect, with resultant heart failure.'

Peasants in the customary blue-grey, pyjama-like costume of modern China shuffled along the corridors of the Chinese hospital I was visiting, undisturbed by the occasional cadres who bore themselves with a greater air of importance. White-coated doctors and nurses dashed from ward to ward. The walls looked creased and battered with constant wear. My senses alone could have told me I was not in the Western hospital in the same city, because there was no acrid, antiseptic odour, only a thick, woody smell of herbs.

I was at home here once again, for this was the kind of place I had chosen for study years before, in another part of China. On this day I was privileged to have an appointment with Dr Lu, the venerable head of the out-patients' department. His name was a legend and his time sought by hundreds of patients and practitioners.

Like queues for soccer matches, lines of prospective patients would start forming before dawn, for the chance of seeing Dr Lu. They came for ordinary coughs, stomach upsets and flu as well as for chronic conditions for which there was no easy answers in Western, or modern, medicine. Why do they come for the simple problems? The only answer they can give is: 'this method works better.'

The chronic conditions were those familiar to any doctor in a developed country: arthritis, hypertension, life-threatening tumours, long-standing difficulties with digestion, elimination of waste or sexual matters, low back pains, menstrual problems, intractable skin conditions, and undefinable nervousness or anxiety. Other complaints were unusual ones – a black coating on the tongue, sweating on one side of the body, strange odours in the armpits. When I asked them, they told me freely that they had been to the Western hospital before, and that the queue was no different there. The only distinction they made was that scientific medicine seemed to work faster, but when it didn't work they soon moved back to the old-style healers.

On our rounds I asked Dr Lu for his opinion about the merits of the two medicines. In a way he was similar to most scientific physicians, for he was aware only of the East–West contrast, but was unfamiliar with other Eastern medicines, such as Indian practice. He struggled at first, straining to make clear his position to a Wester-

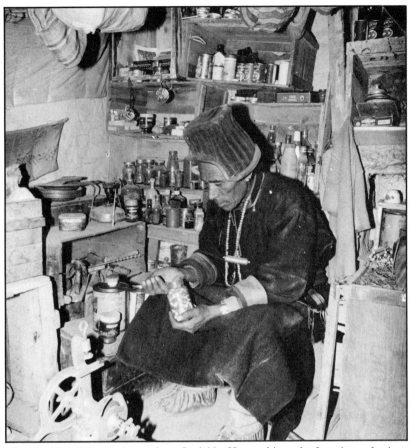

The *Amchi*, a Tibetan doctor from Ladakh. He combines the functions of priest, pharmacist and physician, and treats his patients with a mixture of common sense and traditional medicine

ner. At last he ventured, 'They are like chopsticks and a bowl – two ways of getting at the rice. Modern China needs both. Sometimes the sticks can probe deeper. At other times the embracing bowl fills the need. But in fact both methods serve each other.' He was emphasising the current Chinese policy of uniting modern and traditional practices. More details, I insisted. His answer was honest: 'When surgery or drugs can resolve the problem decisively, that is the best choice. That's the direct, linear, probing line. But when they're not available, or when diagnosis is elusive, the softer, embracing, circular style of our traditional medicine may be better.' And then he added a caveat: 'Never forget that individual patients are always capable of unexpected responses.'

17

I seized upon that enigmatic distinction that comes up so often in East–West comparisons. What did he mean by 'linear' as opposed to 'circular' medical styles? His answer opened up the heart of the dialogue: 'Linear means going right to the problem – detecting it, isolating it, controlling it and usually destroying it. The problem is an invasion, a defect, an aberration: in that view the problem is separate from the person.' So I said that 'circular' must mean dealing with the totality of the person, a person who cannot be cut up into parts. 'Yes,' he said, 'a whole being.'

One can read this distinction a hundred times and not understand its import. Why? Because we in the West are so conditioned to the logic of the scientific method. It works in analysing a carburettor – why not a heart? Is it really possible that a balance of forces within the body – a balance of fire/wind or whatever – can be more important than, or as important as, or at least important to, a specific diagnosis of an infection or hypertension?

Dr Lu insisted that there was only one illness – a disturbance of the balanced way. I knew what it meant to work to restore the harmony of a patient. I had seen all kinds throughout my professional life. The key question that I have had to ask is what sort of patient is before me. Some were meek, some assertive; some were pudgy, some lanky; some slow, some quick. One wears a sweater on warm days, another a T-shirt on blustery mornings. Loud, clear voices, then soft, low voices. I was forced by some feel I was doing them a favour; others demanded a justification for my actions. I see the yin and yang of a patient as the texture of his being – as the Chinese call these bipolar contrasts in nature at large. Yin and yang are neither material entities nor mythical concepts: they are simply ways of organising observations and describing qualities. The distinctions multiply until we realise that even the weight of the bodily organs can vary from one person to the next by a factor of twenty. How much greater must be the distinctive human differences between one person and the next.

Dr Lu's first patient was a young mother with a lifelong history of bronchial asthma. She spoke with a slight wheezing and shortness of breath. As she 'presented' herself to Dr Lu for the first time, she spelt out a familiar tale. Twelve years ago, after a feverish attack, she had entered a Western hospital in order to get through the night. Thereafter she had been cursed with respiratory trouble at every turn: cold or dampness in the weather, difficult or unpleasant household chores, or anything unexpected occurring in her life. Her out-patients' clinic at the Western hospital checked her regularly and maintained her on broncho-dilators, but she had become increasingly sensitive and weak. The drugs she was receiving only put a lid on a continuing problem.

The drugs owe their origin to the herbal arsenal that the Chinese have always used against asthma: mainly the ephedra twig, which contains alkaloids that are chemical cousins to the aminophylline prescribed at the Western hospital. Dr Lu explained that he had used such herbs, along with acupuncture, for acute wheezing attacks or spasms in the lungs. But now the patient herself must be treated, not just the immediate symptoms, for the drug treatment alone was no longer capable of reversing a downward trend.

Dr Lu recorded his observations aloud to me. The patient seemed weak, tired, pale and slow; yet her discomfort did not affect her relaxed mood. Though overweight, she wore extra clothes to protect herself from the slightest chill. Each answer she gave emphasised her gentle, over-compliant mood. Her appetite was poor and she had persistent phlegm. Finally Dr Lu examined her tongue, which proved to be wet and pale, like a small bog. Her pulse was thin, a mere thread. Dr Lu nodded his head and used those expressions that are fundamental to the Chinese world: the cold-wet *yin* was dominating the hot-dry *yang* aspects of life. The patient was too damp and static. I asked him to elaborate. *Yin* originally meant the shady side of a slope; *yang* was the sunny side. *Yin* qualities are quiescent, nurturing and responsive; *yang* qualities are active, bright and dynamic. Together, for the Chinese, they describe the tension that creates health or illness and even life itself.

Dr Lu's prescription began with a combination of eight herbs that had been effective in dealing with disorders of respiration and digestion – due to cold-wetness – since they had first been recorded in a manual of the late Han dynasty, in about the second century AD. Dr Lu confidently told me that these herbs were known to increase the 'fire' of *yang* that was needed to balance her person. He also prescribed acupuncture to boost this effect. His nutritional advice consisted of a warning against such foods as ice-cream and cucumbers. His 'lifestyle' prescription consisted of meditation, classes which were given at the hospital.

The consultation was now over and I could ask Dr Lu about his prognosis. No, he admitted, the asthma might never be cured, but she would become stronger and would not need drugs to sustain her. I asked in a loaded way if he was treating the person instead of the asthma. Dr Lu immediately responded that the asthma was included in his treatment, but that if her fire and water were balanced the asthma would wither away by itself.

The medicines that both Dr Lu and Dr Rathidevi were practising trace their philosophical roots back to the same era – the fifth century BC. It is for a variety of reasons that I have chosen this period as the one at which to start this book. First, it was a turning point in the history of healing; previously, health and illness had been dealt with primarily in magical terms. Second, this subject forms an excellent beginning for me as a doctor, for it was in reading about this period that my own perspective began to broaden.

Before this time, in India and China sickness was attributed to the displeasure of gods or demons; treatment consisted of exorcism and magical ceremonies. In China, the main health care workers were sorcerers, dressed in bird-like costumes. India's oldest religious text, the *Rigveda*, assigns to specific gods the right to punish sin with sickness and pain.

Throughout much of the ancient world there was a general rejection of the 'witchcraft' vision of medicine in the fifth century BC. Just as the golden age of Greek thought was dawning, so the Confucian and Taoist schools were flowering in China, as were the Upanishad and other schools in India. It was no doubt the humanistic bent of these philosophies that set the tone for their new medicines: 'If we are not yet able to serve man, how can we serve spiritual beings?' Confucius replied to a question about the supernatural. The witchdoctor-like shaman had to go underground, but medicine, like any other deeply ingrained tradition, acceded to the popular consciousness. Thus legend portrays the mythical Yellow Emperor giving China its medicine, and the god Indra revealing India's *Ayurveda*.

The main theme that emerged in Chinese and Indian medical thought from this time onwards was not unlike the 'golden mean' of Greece – balance. Health was to be found inside the body – in a balance of natural forces – and not in supernatural interference or altered states of consciousness. The Taoist perception of the world was one of a continuous interplay of forces – dark to light, cold to hot – the familiar contrast of *yin* and *yang*. These simple terms, so basic to Chinese philosophy, seem foreign in both sound and thought to modern Westerners. They are metaphorical images based on the observed world – not concrete things; and they are not to be confused with our own medical polarities: the regulation of blood sugar and fluids, the alternating flow of oxygen and carbon dioxide in breathing, the push and pull of the thyroid gland.

In any event, the theory of *yin* and *yang* evolved over a period of some twenty-five centuries, beginning, legend has it, with the writings of Fu Hsi in the *I Ching*, or *Book of Changes*. *Yin* and *yang* gradually became the reigning model of medicine and overcame the influence of magic and supernaturalism.

In the Indian tradition, *kapha* balances *pitta* in a similar way. *Kapha*, like *yin*, is seen as stabilising, while *pitta*, like *yang*, is fiery. But the Ayurvedic system also includes a third force, *vata*, to mediate this tension. There is no reason to go more deeply into these systems here, except to note that this attempt to understand nature in terms of opposing forces appears in many ancient civilisations. Magic gave way to rational constructs. For the Greek Empedocles the forces were earth, air, fire and water; while for Hindus ether was a fifth, primordial element. The Chinese also had a variant five-element scenario. These ideas related to world views, of which medicine was only a part.

Through those twenty-five centuries since the first enunciation of these theories of natural, opposing forces, Chinese and Indian medicines have come down to their present-day practitioners virtually intact. The key to both systems is that they are observations of the appearance of life, rather than frontal attacks on particular diseases or even disease states. For Dr Lu the general expression for energy, or for the life force, is *chi*. For Dr Rathidevi it is *prana*. When I asked if *prana* could be detected by some device, she replied that it was measurable only by living beings – and to them it was obvious. The pulse was its most vivid expression. As a practitioner of another balanced way of healing, I knew immediately what she meant: the pulse can tell a physician the significant quality balance of a patient when other signs are confused. Dr Rathidevi reminded me that in the old days 'some physicians oiled their fingers daily to keep their sensitivity refined'.

If the Chinese and Indian medical systems appear relatively simple, this is deceptive. In fact, the complexity of these systems is such that a seventh-century Chinese text discusses 1720 disease states. Siddha, the ancient Tamil language version of Ayurveda, deals with 4492 sicknesses. Dr Rathidevi concluded her summary of every case we discussed by saying, 'Of course, it is much more complicated.' The concept of *yin* and *yang* is easy, but each individual has *yins* within *yangs*. As we in the Western world would say, there are circles within circles.

In our haste to make easy classifications, we also think of the *yin-yang* type of theory of balance as the contribution solely of Chinese and Indian medicine. For a long time after I had returned from my studies in the East I assumed that the West was somehow insensitive to this inner world of man, and had to learn it from the 'mystic' Far East. Then one day a friend who had heard one of my lectures casually remarked that I might be interested in a book by Hippocrates that she was reading. I thought it would be a waste of time. Everyone knew, as far as I was concerned, that only his ethical writings were relevant, and that they contained nothing of practical value. But I did look at the book, and I found something that I had spent four years looking for in China; my journey to the East had led me back to the West.

Without any apparent contact with the civilisations of India and China, about five centuries before the Christian era, the Greeks along the Ionian coast of Asia Minor developed a remarkably similar outlook on man's place in the universe. I have already mentioned Empedocles' theory of the four primary elements and the broad rule of behaviour embodied in the phrase 'moderation in all things'. Born in the middle of that astonishing century, Hippocrates was mankind's first non-magical doctor known by name. 'All diseases have a natural origin,' he declared in the ironically titled *Sacred Diseases*. In his *Ancient Medicine* he railed against 'witch doctors, faith-healers, quacks and charlatans', tracing the beginning of medicine not to the gods but to cumulative experience – noted, recorded and evaluated. Most remarkable of all, Hippocrates adapted the fire, water, earth and air of the Greek cosmological system to the microcosm of man: blood, phlegm, black bile and yellow bile respectively. Each of these 'humours' had a distinct quality and texture. When one of the humours dominated, this was what man called illness. The resemblance between Hippocrates' description of the tension between fire and water and the Chinese theory of *yin* and *yang* is uncanny:

> Now all animals, including man, are composed of things different in power but working together in their use, namely fire and water. Both together these are sufficient for one another and for everything else, but each by itself sufficient neither for itself nor for anything else. . . . Fire can move all things always, while water can nourish all things always. . . . Neither of them can gain complete mastery. . . .

Similarly, the Greek concept of life force, *pneuma*, is literally 'air' – as are the Chinese *chi* and the Hindu *prana*. But we must be cautious of making facile comparisons, for each concept has a distinct cultural flavour. The Chinese *chi* is more material and moving; the Indian *prana* more transcendent and hierarchical; while the Greek *pneuma* has an intelligence and an unfolding quality.

As one would expect, the Greeks also worked out a complete theory of temperament based on the four humours, a theory of vessels or channels to carry them, and even 'bleeding' points that correspond to certain clinical applications of acupuncture. In the Hippocratic system the physician treated the patient with diet, exercise and herbs, always concentrating on the key question: What elemental qualities are out of balance? Is the patient disproportionately sanguine (fire), placid (water), excitable (air) or inhibited (earth)? The Romans took over this system with few modifications, and its major theoreticians, such as Galen, lived in Rome.

If Greek medicine was as effective as the Eastern systems, why did it vanish from Western civilisation? Perhaps the reason can be found in the gradual transcendence of the new ethos of Christianity, in which illness and misfortune were regarded merely as 'things of the world', to be endured as a form of penance in anticipation of the world to come. As St Basil of Caesarea (*fl.* AD 370) preached to his flock: 'Disease is accepted by the just like an athletic contest, in which, by virtue of patience, a great crown is expected.' Many aspects of healing came to be coloured with religious beliefs, as individual saints were appointed guardians over particular diseases and the old sites of pagan healing rites were turned into shrines for healing by miracles. Yet there was one pathway by which Greek medicine has come down to our times.

The fascinating story of this transmission concerns a small but important Christian sect, the Nestorians. In the late fifth century this theological splinter group was pronounced heretical – for their belief in the dominance of the human nature of Jesus – and was forced to flee the Eastern Roman Empire, centred on Constantinople. The Nestorians were given asylum in Persia, in what is now southwest Iran, where they found sympathetic allies in the Persians and Jews of Jundi-Shapur; together the two groups set up the new medical centre of the Western world, translating Greek texts into Syrian, Hebrew and later Arabic. When the Moslems over-ran the city in 636, they recognised the value of the work being done here; graduates of the Jundi-Shapur medical school had treated Mohammed and later the caliphs.

This medical tradition, fertilised by Arabs, Persians and Jews and eventually centred on Baghdad, was reintroduced to Europe in the eleventh century. And so at universities such as Salerno, Padua,

Paris, and Oxford medicine came to be the science of Hippocrates, Galen, the Moslem Avicenna, and Moses Maimonides, the twelfth-century Jewish scholar. The Moslem conquest of India likewise introduced this strain of Greek medicine to the Asian subcontinent, where it is still known to this day by the Arabic word for Greek, Unani.

In the West, however, the medicine of the balanced way came up against an opposing force of an order entirely different from fire and water. It was not until the nineteenth century that someone found a name for it, but its aims were plain. It was science.

In a series of hammer blows from the Renaissance in the mid-sixteenth century to the Age of Reason in the early eighteenth, one after another the tenets of Greek humoral medicine were demolished. Vesalius overthrew Greek anatomical speculation in 1543. In a public lecture in 1616, William Harvey demonstrated the modern concept of the circulation of the blood and so for ever banished ancient notions of humoral movement. In 1625, a colleague of Galileo's, Santorio Santorio, made the remarkable discovery that a person described in Greek medicine as 'hot' or bilious and one described as 'cold' or phlegmatic have the same measured temperature. Since it was Galileo who had lent his friend the thermometer he had invented, he too can claim a place in the history of scientific medicine.

A new principle had been applied to the observation of reality: our senses cannot be trusted. Qualities had to be reduced to quantities, images to lines, speculation to experimentation. The living continuity of experience, the actual texture of human life, was fragmented into the higher truth of mathematics. According to the new science, as elaborated by Francis Bacon and others, the observer must remove himself from the world he is observing and rely on tools of measurement. Reality was reduced to units of space, time, motion and matter. The senses, in Descartes' words, were regarded as 'confused thoughts'. Copernicus' thesis regarding the position of the sun in the centre of the solar system, published in the same year as Vesalius' anatomical studies, showed that man's ordinary experience of a sunrise was an illusion. Though this revolution in scientific thought may seem mundane today, it changed the Western world's vision of reality in a dramatic way.

Nowadays, because of the power of the experimental method, we take it for granted that quantitative science is the port of ultimate knowledge. Yet an important part of the reality of people's lives consists of just those things that are illusory or secondary to science. Not everything can be reduced to repeatable experiments, least of all the life of colours and sounds, pleasures and pains, ambitions and purposes. It is equally tempting but fallacious to try to reduce health care to thermometers and electrocardiograms, to X-rays and microscopes – in running from the sensory world to embrace science we have abandoned some of our humanity.

My mind went back again to that hospital complex in Madras where I had met Dr Rethidevi. As I have said, by the early nineteenth century the Greek version of the balanced way had vanished from the universities of Europe. But here, in another ward of the Arignar Anna Hospital, one can observe physicians in the usual white coats practising the medicine of the Greeks – Unani. They are still balancing humours. The works of Galen, Avicenna and Maimonides are not relegated to the rare book shelves in the library, but are in the ward and are referred to daily in clinical application. Hippocrates, the father of medicine, is looked to for guidance not in Manhattan or Harley Street, but in a crowded clinic in central Madras.

I made it my business to see at first hand how this ancient medicine was practised. The doctor, or *hakim*, in charge of the Unani in-patients' and out-patients' wards, Syed Imanunddin Ahmed, was a handsome young man who had graduated from the government Unani medical school ten years earlier. I asked if Moslems alone came to see him. 'Ask my patients,' he responded with a smile. They were equally divided between Moslems and Hindus, Christians or atheists, and they came because they had heard that it worked.

I noticed a patient with vitiligo, a skin disease that, to the lay person, resembles leprosy. She had come here because the blemishes made it impossible for a woman to marry, and the doctors at the Western hospital had told her that the only available treatment was in Unani medicine. She happily showed me how much smaller the markings were after a few weeks of treatment here.

In the next room, a woman with jaundice was more talkative because her English was excellent. She had been told to come to the Unani section by her aunt, who had recovered from hepatitis here. The yellow colour was going away quickly, she told me.

Hakim Ahmed was enthusiastic about Unani medicine. Nine generations of his family had been doctors, and all his brothers and cousins were graduates of the local Unani medical school. I pointed out to him the irony of a Westerner having to learn about the heritage of Hippocrates from a Madras doctor, but Hakim Ahmed found it only mildly amusing, for he had had numerous encounters with sceptics from other cultures.

2·THE·MYSTERY· OF·ILLNESS

On his deathbed in 1895 Louis Pasteur is reputed to have said, in reference to his lifelong rivalry with Claude Bernard, 'Bernard was right. Microbes are nothing, the soil is everything.' Coming from the man who proved the existence of germs, this is a startling thought in its modernity; it is relevant to the issue of illness, as perceived by patients, and to the subject of disease, as perceived by modern doctors. By their very nature these doctors deal with bits and pieces – microbes, hormone deficiencies or tumours – while patients experience illness as the disorder, disruption and possibly disintegration of their ordinary lives. It is a division that has existed for as long as there have been doctors who name diseases, and the contrast only becomes sharper in the consulting rooms of scientific doctors. In order to understand the multiplicity and aptness of all the healing arts, we must first ask what illness is all about – how does the actual person perceive it?

The Jewish Talmud, an under-utilised source of insight, has much to say about the mystery of illness. Who determines if a man is too sick to observe the solemn Day of Atonement fast? The Talmud says that even if a hundred doctors think it unnecessary to violate this sacred law, the patient alone must decide, because 'the heart knoweth its own bitterness' better than anyone else. There is a threshold of tolerance, outside the gaze of any physician, that can only be private and personal.

Various types of research confirm the Talmud's point of view. In a random sample of 1000 adults living in London, less than 5 per cent showed no symptoms of illness during a two-week period. Of the 95 per cent who experienced discomfort or abnormalities, only 20 per cent saw a doctor; almost another 20 per cent took no action whatsoever; and well over 50 per cent took some sort of action that did not involve a doctor. People choose to see doctors for reasons that bear no relation to the incidence of maladies in the population at large.

Another study undertaken in London showed that if a person had chest pain the odds were 1 in 14 that he or she would consult a doctor, while a change in energy would impel only 1 in 456 to do so. Someone with backache is twice as likely to go to the doctor as a person with digestive disturbance. Other community-wide surveys confirmed these findings: the person decides what constitutes a patient.

When a person finally decides to see a doctor, it is doubtful that he or she can explain why. In *Socio-medical Enquiries*, a readable book despite its forbidding title, the Boston sociologist Irving Kenneth Zola summarises much of the research on how people make what can be a costly and often time-consuming decision. It seems that people react to symptoms of illness in remarkably different ways; for example, most people continually exhibit at least one symptom that alone impels some individuals to make their way to the doctor's surgery. To put it another way, there is widespread physical discomfort but little perceived illness. A doctor typically sees only a small and unrepresentative sample of people's complaints.

Among the reasons people give for seeking medical help are the newness of a symptom, recognition of a habitual problem or the observation of others with similar complaints. The alchemy of change to the vulnerable, fearful and fragile state of patienthood can be mysterious.

I find it essential in my own medical practice to discover why a patient has finally decided to see me. In non-emergencies, after a few exploratory questions and the recital of the patient's story I simply ask: Why now? Strangely, this question is seldom asked by most practitioners I have encountered. It is the type of question about personal background that is noticeably absent even in Chinese medicine with its emphasis on observable appearances and sensations.

That particular question opens many doors. Rarely do I hear something like 'I couldn't bear it any longer.' People seem to have their ailments for a long time, and it is usually something extraneous to what we would call 'health' that brings them to the doctor. The migraine starts interfering with a musical rehearsal; the stomach pains make it difficult to go out for beers with the lads; now that the secret lover has gone the person doesn't mind the prospect of going to hospital. Why the delay? In the USA it may be money – but the patient has no more now than he or she had, say, a year ago; the children may have needed the attention – but they're still around; it may have been a dislike or fear of doctors – but that feeling hasn't changed now. What brings them to the doctor is as much the music,

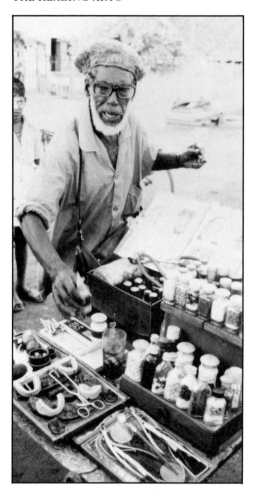

Throughout the world, before most people go to doctors they try home remedies, local advice and folk healers. This is a street 'doctor' in India, with cures for everything from dental problems to lack of fertility

their friends or a new situation as the discomfort. If I find the experiential reason I know I am on to something that may help me heal the person.

One's immediate concerns can distract one from the perception of illness. In the heat of the game a footballer may not immediately notice quite a severe injury, but he will probably seek out the physiotherapist if he feels the slightest twinge in his knee while training. Symptoms, too, can have special and personal memories for each individual and can speed the transition from ordinary person to patient. A mild cough may remind a man of his grandfather's tuberculosis; a drop of blood from haemorrhoids has greater impact if your sister died of bowel cancer.

The social and historical milieu can shape the boundary between illness and health. Various social groups ignore discomfort simply because they are commonplace. If it is perceived as part of life, it is not sickness. Afghans accept diarrhoea, steel-mill workers are resigned to backaches, some African tribes think nothing of hallucinations, and contemporary young women consider it normal to have painful periods. We may laugh at our ancestors for thinking that not having an illness is a sign of ill health: children in the Middle Ages, for example, were regarded as ill if they did not have mild eczema, and some tribes in South America and southern Africa would not allow their young men to marry until they had contracted certain skin conditions or malaria. Yet in our own era we now know that having modified polio as a child is protective against the crippling form of the disease that occurs in young adults. And German measles is welcomed for a little girl as a precaution against catching the same disease in her child-bearing years. Early illness, in short, may mean health later in life.

Illness can have its cultural or national hallmark. A French-woman announces she is suffering from a *crise de foie* – she has overworked her liver with too much rich food and feels a need to cleanse her system with mineral waters. Or a Malaysian 'runs amok' in an illness unique to that people – dashing into the street brandishing a knife. Cultural differences dictate the Englishman's self-prescription for what is called a 'chill': 'Feed a cold and starve a fever.' In China, I regularly treated patients whose problem was 'fear of cold', but I have yet to have one such patient in the United States.

Consider how our ethnic origins shape our experience of illness. A native American Indian child is often taught from an early stage to ignore pain, whereas an adored Italian baby boy might be expected to register the least malaise to his mother. Thus childhood conditioning can stay with one into adulthood. Mark Zborowski, in his classic anthropological study of a hospital for ex-servicemen in New York City, demonstrated that Protestant 'Old Americans', Irish, Italians and Jews have marked differences in pain behaviour and attitudes. Ethnic origins can give the bitterness of sickness its own special taste. The Old American patient tended to be detached, precise and rational: 'The leg hurts', never '*My* leg hurts.' Pain was a warning signal to bring him to a doctor who had the 'proper credentials' to alleviate the underlying sickness. He didn't want his ailment to interfere in the doctor's performance of his duties. The Irishman outwardly resembled the Old American but his inner world was different. He wasn't concerned about the pain; he could 'suffer alone', but dreaded 'not being able to work'. Often a member of his family had to drag him to receive medical attention, and he was sceptical about doctors anyway. The Italian complained freely, drawing attention to his pain with groans, moans and tears. He wanted immediate relief from pain; discomfort interfered with his social life. When the pain was relieved by analgesics, he was back to his normal self. He trusted the doctor because he had a likeable personality. The Jewish patient, like the Italian, displayed his feelings freely, using dramatic vocabulary. But he often secretly hid his analgesics; his preoccupation was the cause and significance of the pain, not relief of the symptom. He shopped around for his doctor, consulting several, and reserved the final decision for himself. Health, he thought, was an exception, a temporary lapse between extended periods of sickness.

Zborowski's study may seem like racist stereotyping, but a patient, and especially a doctor, unaware of how ethnic origins shape the boundaries of illness, can cause and compound serious health problems. An Old American may try to be too accommodating to the doctor and actually hurt himself; an Irishman may need to be probed more deeply to find out what is being experienced; an Italian may too easily give up being a patient, leading to future problems; and a Jew who does not have his personal concerns taken into consideration may not comply with the treatment. Though each ethnic group may have the same protruding spinal disc or constricted blood vessels, the patient's experience and needs must be approached differently.

So a definition of illness is not easy. Even when our powerful diagnostic tools are brought to bear on biomedical disease, illness is elusive. What is observed as osteo-arthritis on an X-ray may never be experienced as pain by the patient. Sometimes an autopsy reveals a cancer which should have registered severe illness but was unnoticed by the person. The microscope cannot discern when disease is illness. An article in *Paediatrics*, 1962, reported how one hundred persons in 16 families agreed to have throat swabs taken and cultured every three weeks in addition to times of acute illness. Researchers found that 20 per cent showed 'strep throat' – streptococcal infection – but in less than half these cases did the scientific disease mean any illness of the patient. Preventative medicine calls for early detection of such diseases as hypertension, diabetes and cancer – and for the most part this is laudable. But sometimes one wonders about the patient who is pushed over the border of pain and patienthood by being told of his disease, when he might have been better off without this intrusion. It is not uncommon for the side effects of drugs that are used to reduce high blood pressure in the elderly to present more problems than if the hypertension were left untreated. High blood pressure is an example of that curious phenomenon of the communication of news sometimes being as dangerous as what that news announces: in a Canadian study, reported in the *New England Journal of Medicine* in 1978, it was shown that absenteeism doubled when workers were informed of their hypertension.

Eric J. Cassel, also writing in the *New England Journal of Medicine*, told a similar story of how the name alone of a disease can increase illness. A woman with presumed sciatic pain was relieved with small doses of codeine; when the doctor subsequently told her that the diagnosis was actually cancer, massive amounts of codeine could not cope with the pain.

While this cancer patient may well have needed treatment, all medical systems share an unfortunate tendency to want to 'cure' conditions that may not always be dangerous or abnormal. Somehow, doctors trust what they call abnormality or intrusion more than what the patient experiences. Chiropractors will straighten spines and Chinese doctors harmonise pulses, all creating illness where there is only the appearance of disease. This is especially true with the plethora of modern medical diagnostic techniques. Tonsils were once removed automatically in the United States, and numerous other operations from circumcision to appendicectomy were rationalised on preventive grounds. But the conclusions of modern medicine change so fast that even the specialist has trouble keeping track of the latest 'truth'. At a recent meeting of the American Diabetes Association, a speaker asked for a show of hands on the carbohydrate-restriction regimen that has been in vogue for diabetics since the 1930s. Virtually everyone agreed that this was still the recommended procedure. The speaker then pointed out that the literature had been recommending the opposite strategy for at least four years. The speaker wryly reminded his audience – all specialists in diabetes – that it was Galen who, noticing that flies were attracted to the urine of diabetics, guessed that the patients were in need of more carbohydrates to compensate for this observable loss of sugar. That was in the first century AD.

Another notorious episode in the management of diabetes underlines the difficulty of drawing a line between sickness and health.

Noting that diabetics in several American hospitals for ex-servicemen seemed to show improvement with a reduction in medications, including insulin, the director of the hospitals redefined the diabetics under his care to exclude those who no longer needed high doses of insulin. After this edict, of course, the patients were just as ill or as healthy as before; critics made much of the fact that the disease had been halved by a stroke of a pen.

While the forces that make illness can vary from ethnic background to the meaning of words, even the forces that make physical disease can defy simple classification and include almost any type of life event. Studies have shown that one is more likely to develop a disease after any stressful event, and in close correlation with the seriousness of the stress. A study of 5000 British widowers published in *The Lancet* in 1963 showed that disease rates increased 40 per cent in the first six months after their wife's death. A recent report from Mount Sinai School of Medicine in New York City showed that the T cells and lymphocytes, important parts of the immunological response, underwent pathological changes in bereaved husbands of cancer patients. A study of twenty-five cases of full-blown diabetes, none of whom had had previous symptoms, showed that twenty persons had suffered severe setbacks shortly before onset. A special government medical task force investigating the determining factors for surviving atherosclerotic heart disease in Massachusetts reported that the most reliable prognosticator for surviving heart disease was not non-smoking, normal blood pressure, or low cholesterol levels but 'job satisfaction'. The second-best indication was 'overall happiness'. A nine-year study, reported in the *American Journal of Epidemiology*, made in Alameda County, California, of 4700 men and women showed that people who lacked social and community ties were more likely to fall sick and die.

Even invading microbes are affected by everything that affects our lives. Doctors at the Vienna Neurological Clinic hypnotised subjects at various times to either a joyous state or a sad state. Blood serum taken when they were happy clumped typhoid bacilli much more quickly than blood at sad times. Six hundred employees at a United States Army base were given psychological tests during the summer. The twenty-six who reported to the infirmary during the winter with flu (nineteen diagnosed by virus isolation) divided into two groups: those who got well in less than fourteen days and those who were sick for more than twenty-one days. The decisive factor, according to the summer tests, was a tendency to 'have the blues' and not feel good about oneself. In *The Social Causes of Illness*, Richard Totman summarises the recent research on the stress–psychology–disease connection by concluding that it involves a mechanism that is a factor in virtually every disease.

Interestingly enough, when we finally do acknowledge illness our first movement is not to a healer. There is one country in the world in which three out of four people who feel discomfort do not see a doctor. That country is not in the Third World; it is Britain, with its National Health Service. And, despite the number of facilities in the United States, the same is true there also.

The reason is simple: self-medication is the dominant healing practice of the West, as it always has been anywhere. Television advertisements are its newest source of information and the chemist's shop (or, as it is more pointedly known in the USA, the drug store) its source of supply. In addition there is a regular exchange of drugs and medicines among relatives and neighbours. Recently vitamins, special diets, herbs and exercise regimes have been added to this amateur medical bazaar. Advice is dispensed from these people as well as from strangers who have experienced a similar illness. Arthur Kleinman of Harvard estimates that between 70 and 90 per cent of healing in the industrialised nations originates from these sources. The percentage is higher in the Third World. The situation reminds one of the tradition that in ancient Babylon the sick would wait at the city gate for advice from someone who admitted to having had the same malady cured.

Too often this new folk medicine, like old folk medicine, does not work and the person concerned is forced either to live with it or to seek professional advice. The inner voice, the 'bitterness of the heart', leads one in that direction. The Talmud, in fact, prescribes as one of the necessary conditions of life to live in the vicinity of a doctor.

What is his or her role? On the surface it seems to be the elimination or relief of perceived discomfort, deformity or disability. But actually it is something more. The pain of childbirth (at least until recently) or that of a medieval Christian flagellant did not expect a medical response. Chinese women never had their crippled bound feet treated by Chinese doctors. And the advanced elderly people who can only move with the most halting of steps do not seek a doctor's aid for their disability. Going to the healer means trying to change the perceived *disorder* in the way of things.

When a patient goes to a scientific doctor, the healer is most comfortable if the patient's disruption can be located in a concrete, physical and isolatable place. Using some discussion, but relying mainly on technology, the biomedical doctor gazes into the body concealed behind the skin and can detect even the smallest molecules. The invisible, material and mindless determinants of reality are revealed.

The Chinese physician, as we have seen, uses a different approach. He takes great pains to observe the patient's appearance, movements and pulse. In what is visible and sensory he sees manifestations of the invisible forces of nature.

In Nigeria native doctors or *babalawaos* do not bother with the patient's story. Instead, the patient whispers into a handful of palm nuts. The *babalawao* casts the nuts like dice, and from their position divines the reason for illness. For the African witchdoctor, the invisible forces of the spirits, imagination and will impinge on man. All parts of the universe exist in a state of interdependence. In an altered state of consciousness, the healer can read these forces in the nuts just as the cardiologist can read an electrocardiogram.

Notice how the assigning of a name to illness, unless it has the cruel meaning of something like cancer, can give a form of relief. You've now pinned it down, and can't wait to start the medication or

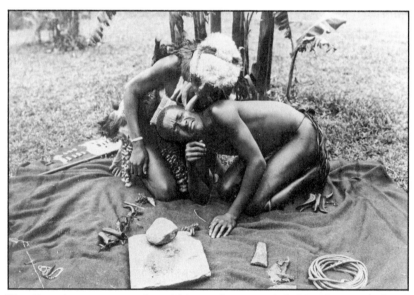

The *Sanusi*, or surgeon, of an African tribe, surrounded by the practical and magical instruments of his art. He is performing a ceremonial bloodletting, an *Ukulumeka*, using an ox-horn. Whatever is used,the healer is the mediator between the disturbed universe of the patient and the intact universe of the healthy person

treatment. The doctor's admonition to come back in a few days' time places you firmly under his or her wing. All this is part of the response to illness and the beginning of the healing process. And all this works to one degree or another, whatever the particular school of healing of the doctor. He or she may be scientific, or oriental, or a jack of all trades; all that matters is that the healer should reconnect you in one way or another with the coherent, well-behaved world in which people are healthy.

Yes, you say, but doesn't the scientific doctor know more about the real causes of illnesses and their appropriate cures? This question must be carefully examined. First, it is an undisputed fact that the paraphernalia of modern medicine is awe-inspiring. Within the lifetime of many people we have gone from the days when the doctor's bag contained little more than a tongue depressor and a stethoscope to a time when neurotransmitters can be tracked in our brains by nuclear magnetic resonance. Yet the chronic diseases – heart disease, cancer, diabetes; the ones that will kill us – still largely elude the scientific net; and many diseases that ruin our lives, such as arthritis, allergies and depression, continue to haunt us. Studies have shown that half of the population of hospitals are incurable. The power of the scientific approach lies in the reduction of things to their elementary parts, which can be dealt with independently. But degenerative and chronic disease cannot easily be cured by this sort of split vision. As René Dubos writes, in *Mirage of Health*, 'Search for *the* causes may be a hopeless pursuit because most disease states are the direct outcome of a constellation of circumstances rather than the direct result of single determinant factors.'

Then there is the changeable nature of science – both a curse and a blessing. Scientific medicine can react rapidly to change; by contrast, some Eastern medicines can change only minutely over centuries. On the other hand, this has the unfortunate consequence that scientific medicine is often erratic. For example, it was once considered a doctor's task to reduce the fever of anyone who saw him; now the theory seems to be that fevers should be allowed to run their course as part of the body's innate defence mechanism. Someone finally discovered that there was no evidence in the general population of brain damage or any other untoward results of fever; in fact, it may even help to cure infections. We were once told to clean our ears with swabs or have them cleaned with warm oil and elaborate syringes; now many doctors advise a gentle massage of the ear lobe and cleaning with the tip of one's forefinger! Much more distressing

35

is the result of a 1985 US Government study involving eighty-nine institutions and thousands of breast cancer patients. The results indicate that most women with early stages of this disease can just as well be treated by small-scale surgery, called lumpectomies, as by the complete removal of the breast. This means that of the approximately 100,000 American women likely to develop breast cancer in 1986, most are unlikely to be candidates of drastic disfigurement as their counterparts were in 1984.

Because we have all experienced the uncertainties of being a patient and the relief of healing, we assume that modern medicine has found the causes of disease and thus is responsible for the extension of our lives and our sense of being well. Yet this is a widespread fallacy on two levels. First, because of the placebo effect and other aspects of the healing process – which I will call 'mythical' for the moment – a high percentage of illness is relieved regardless of medications; merely seeing a professional initiates results. Second, and more important, the provision of adequate food, clean water and proper sanitation has reduced or eliminated the great killer diseases throughout the world independently of modern drugs. The mortality rate from tuberculosis in Britain dropped from 400 per 100,000 people in 1840 to 200 in 1880 (two years before the TB bacillus was discovered) to only 50 in 1950 – just before the drugs arrived to give TB the *coup de grâce*. These drugs can only cure when the environment is properly administered; they have not affected the incidence of TB in those countries where living conditions are similar to those of nineteenth-century Britain. Most of the other dreaded infectious diseases of the last century disappeared because of life-style and environmental changes as did leprosy and bubonic plague in earlier centuries.

Nor are the methods of modern medicine the most proven ones. As the epidemiologist Archibald Cochrane has demonstrated in *Effectiveness and Efficiency*, the vast majority of currently accepted clinical procedures have never been subjected to critical examination by randomised controlled clinical trials. And even when such work is carried out, the results are inconclusive or worse. Cochrane's formidable and extensive survey ranges from a study showing that oral anti-diabetic therapy is less valuable than diet control, to one revealing that acute heart patients treated at home do as well as patients treated in coronary care units.

This is not meant to decry the value of antibiotics, which accelerated the decline of infections, or of other achievements of modern medicine such as the spectacular interventions of surgery. Rather, it is meant to put scientific medicine's achievement in a realistic perspective. The other healing arts are not necessarily better, just different. I know from first-hand experience that each of the other healing arts suffers from the inherent limitations of its finite tools of diagnosis and treatment. Our criticism of modern medicine applies to other forms of medicine too. The unbridled population growth of China is the result not of the success of Chinese medicine, but of improved living conditions and the lingering tradition of large families as a form of life insurance. The ancient Chinese were as prone as Westerners to overdo a good thing. They searched for longevity in the alchemical branch of their medicine, but improved mortality rates eluded them. This was partly because most of their alchemist potions included the red stone cinnabar, which contains mercury and turns out to be an insidious poison. And Nigerian witchdoctors have caused more than one inadvertent cardiac arrest. Arrogance does not reside with modern medical practitioners alone.

When a person is ill, the imperative to heal is great. The Talmud tells us that doctors can break any law, such as the Sabbath law of rest, to treat compelling illness. But there is no single system of medicine that can encompass illness, or even disease, in its infinite forms and its unplumbed depths. Stephanus, a sixth-century Greek doctor, understood this dilemma implicitly when he said that medicine suffered from a fundamental contradiction: its theory grasps universals only, while its practice deals with individuals. No two men are alike, he continued; the differences are 'ineffable and cannot be subjected to concepts'. Every healing art sees illness in its own terms. Patients need to remember that the illness is theirs and theirs alone. The Talmud says that in God's vision there is no difference between saving an individual life and saving the entire world. The implication is that not only is life precious, but each unique life is as complex and impenetrable as the entire cosmos. Once we awaken from the dogmatic slumber of believing that one medicine has all the answers, then we can go on with an open mind to examine the whole range of healing systems that the genius of the human race has so patiently worked out.

3·HANDS·ON

Perhaps the greatest loss that medicine has suffered over the course of the centuries is that of personal contact. Sophisticated doctors throughout the world tend to avoid the healing power of the human hand. The only form of contact that seems to have survived worldwide is the elevated art of surgery – perhaps because it can be practised in the most detached and impersonal setting. Other types of physical contact are dispersed into secondary, often disparaged categories, which are left to vie among themselves for some badge of accomplishment: osteopathy, chiropractic, acupuncture, bone-setting and manipulation and massage in its many forms.

Yet the power of touch is recognised universally, from new childbirth techniques to 'crisis' psychiatry. It is always an intense moment when a strange hand first touches us, when we allow some-one to penetrate our defensive *cordon sanitaire*. Body language is direct yet subtle, capable of expressing even in a handshake a whole gamut of emotions from love to aggression. A doctor's hands move cautiously yet expressively over the person on the examination table, and his ability to give a reassuring pat on the back or upper arm after the task is complete can elevate him or her from a mere technician to a physician in the full sense of the word.

Far from being able to exude a feeling of fellowship and warmth, in many societies doctors, especially men, have assumed the mantle of an unapproachable priesthood. Worse, the profession condemns some, and discourages many, of the therapies of touch that have helped millions of people physically as well as psychologically. From the perspective of other cultures and other times such attitudes could politely be described as provincial.

In the Ebers Smith Papyrus, which dates from the earliest period of Egyptian history, the most common phrase referred to the use of hands in therapy. Archaeological evidence indicates that massage was used at least twenty-five centuries ago in China to alleviate urinary retention. Among tribal people massage has always been called on to help expel demons, or just to make one feel good. The famous Greek doctor Asclepiades regularly rubbed the vertebral column of his patients in the treatment of various illnesses. By this period in history, the first century BC, there is ample evidence for the widespread practice of massage.

It is a reasonable speculation that the probing of the body and its orifices with the fingers cautiously preceded surgery, and records of ancient surgery are almost frightening in their variety and universality. It is also tempting to see the rise of surgery in recent times as the death knell of many of the other manipulative arts, which could not compete with the glamour and the immediacy of the scalpel. In any event, surgery is clearly the most intrusive and drastic healing art, and is extensively recognised and utilised. It is mentioned here partly for the contrast it exhibits with those therapies demanding interaction with the patient.

The very term 'surgery' derives from the Greek words for 'hand work'. Stone Age tools were made of sharpened flint, and skulls from that era have been discovered which show signs of having undergone the difficult operation of trepanning, the surgical opening of the skull usually performed to relieve pressure on the brain. The fact that many skulls show evidence of multiple operations and regrowth of tissue implies a reasonable rate of success – yet this procedure was considered quite dangerous a century ago. In other early civilisations, including African ones, it is clear that such operations as amputations, caesarian sections, tonsillectomies, removal of bladder stones and even plastic surgery were quite feasible. The ancient Hindu surgeon, Susruta, used 125 different surgical instruments. The Hippocratic writings discuss several surgical procedures, as well as aligning dislocations, fractures and skeletal derangements.

Between the time of Celsus, who excised tumours and patched hernias in the first century AD, and the coming of anaesthesia and antiseptics in the mid-nineteenth century, surgery was at best a desperate gamble. The premier position we accord it today would astonish the practitioners of the Middle Ages, who were relegated to the status of barbers.

The art of acupuncture, which has developed for about 2500 years, may also have been preceded by a sort of finger massage, the spontaneous reaction of touch and warmth applied to an injured part of the body. This unique contribution of the Chinese likewise had its gruesome moments, but it is more of an art rather than a coarse intervention in an inert body. The Chinese have a theory that the vital life force (*chi*) requires an internal 'aqueduct' system merely to allow the body to function. Although the Indians postulated a similar network of channels, they did not pursue this thought to the logical conclusion of acupuncture: that these 'meridians' might have juncture points along their length that would be sensitive to manipulation. Perhaps the Chinese model of only fifty-nine meridians (fourteen being clinically important) was more workable; the Hindu system contemplated 700. Nevertheless, in the Indian Ayurvedic system there was once a strong emphasis on *marma*, the massage of more than a hundred points on the skin. While *marma* has faded in importance, acupuncture has enjoyed a renaissance in the West, spurred on by the reopening of US–Chinese relations in the 1970s.

As in Chinese medicine as a whole, the theory of acupuncture comes back to the balancing of the opposing forces of *yin* and *yang*. Classically, there are 365 juncture points where this 'switching' can take place. Over the centuries, more points have been added, but the theory is the same: finger massage, heat stimulation or the insertion of very fine needles at those points can affect potential imbalances along each meridian or in the body.

It has taken centuries of trial and error, with much speculation, to suggest which pressure points influence the multiplicity of possible imbalances in this complicated, interwoven network. In virtually every case of illness, it is thought there is a combination of points which must be touched simultaneously to bring about the desired change.

The apparatus of first-rate acupuncture (for there are variations in quality in any art) is as precisely designed for the penetration of the body as are any surgeon's instruments. Once made of bronze, copper, tin, gold or silver, needles nowadays are hair-like slivers of stainless steel. They produce only a slight twinge upon insertion, whether to a depth of a millimetre or two at the fingertips or 3–4 inches in the buttocks. Individual sessions may last for thirty minutes or so, and courses of treatment for several weeks or even longer in cases of chronic illness.

There is a natural temptation to try to relate the results of acupuncture to the anatomical theories of modern medicine. As I have suggested already, it would be equally improper to attempt to justify a tenet of scientific medicine by examining the extent to which it conformed to, let us say, Indian medicine. I would emphasise here that Chinese or Indian or even shaman medicine is as logical as

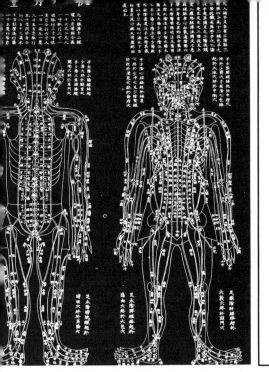

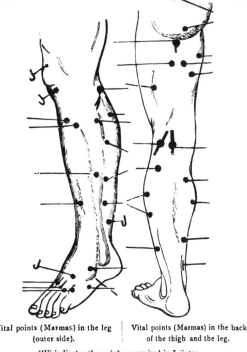

Vital points (Marmas) in the leg
(outer side).

Vital points (Marmas) in the back
of the thigh and the leg.

"J" indicates the points recognised in Juijutsu.

Left. Even the oldest charts of meridians and acupuncture points demonstrate the precision and depth of knowledge that lie behind the insertion of needles to alter the internal balance of a patient

Right. Indian vital points, *marmas*, on the legs. They can be treated for healing, must be avoided in traditional surgery, and were points of attack in the martial arts

scientific medicine; each examines a different facet of the same person and an attempt to deal directly with his suffering. But if the conceit of superiority can be put aside, it is interesting to see how acupuncture and Western medical theories can converge on some points.

Perhaps the insertion of needles stimulates the release of endorphins, those neurotransmitters that act like morphine. Or the needles may produce an anaesthetic effect by jamming the lower nerve bundles in the central nervous system, causing more stimulus, in effect, than the system can handle. Experienced acupuncturists welcome this sort of dialogue, but insist that it has only a little to do with the multitude of clinical applications unrelated to pain-killing.

And so we come back to the feature of hands on the body in relation to healing. Doctors are now recognising that physical contact is crucial during the early stages of life. In fact, the skin is the largest and most sensitive bodily organ. It was discovered some years ago in a maternity hospital in Bogotá, Colombia, that premature babies, who could not be afforded the luxury of protective glass capsules like their counterparts in richer countries, survived quite well in a sling between their mothers' breasts. The practice is spreading to Britain: it was an inexpensive form of temperature control and, not surprisingly, it made mothers happier. This 'tenderness phenomenon' was described in the 1950s: institutionalised infants became emaciated when they did not receive caressing touches.

What is surprising about such reports is that they seem naïve. The salutary results of close personal contact permeate Western literature. After Captain Cook set foot on Tahiti in 1777 he wrote:

> I returned on board with Otoo's mother, his three sisters, and eight more women. At first I thought they came into my boat with no other view than to get passage . . . but when they got to the ship they told me that had come to cure me of the disorder that I complained of, which was a sort of rheumatic pain in one side from my hip to my foot. I was desired to lay down in the midst of them, then as many as could get round me began to squeeze me with both hands from head to foot, but more especially the parts where the pain was, till they made my bones crack and a perfect mummy of my flesh . . . in short after being under their hands about a quarter hour I was glad to get away from them. However I found immediate relief from the operation. They gave me another rubbing down before I went to bed and I found myself pretty easy all the night after. They repeated the operation the next morning before they went ashore, and again in the evening when they came on board, after which I found the pains intirely removed.

Anyone who has ever suffered from sciatic pain running down a leg will be envious of Captain Cook. Yet there is nothing in this description of his sensations that would be much different from what is experienced under the hands of a modern osteopath or chiropractor.

Massage and manipulation are so common in the Far East that no one pays much attention to them; people suffering from no particular pain go for a massage just because they feel like it. It is practised regularly within families, especially on babies. In China it has always been a trade for the blind, who are taught in special schools. As we have seen, it is an important feature of Ayurvedic medicine in India: the masseur often works herbs into the skin while, for example, cooling coconut oil is poured over the patient's forehead. In Japan the techniques can be equally elaborate, involving pressure on acupuncture points (shiatsu) or manipulation by teachers of martial arts, who often double as doctors.

With few exceptions, in Western countries the healing technique of manipulation and massage has long been considered a second-rate one – at best exotic, at worst bizarre, superstitious or immoral. This attitude can perhaps be traced to the influence of religion: at the Council of Trent in 1563 both surgery and the manipulation of the vertebrae were denounced. In the Middle Ages, the expulsion of demons was indeed believed by many to coincide with the click of the back or neck.

Yet the practice of both arts continued. Some healers, such as Ambroise Paré, the only French Protestant spared by Charles IX during the gruesome Massacre of St Bartholomew's Eve in 1572, actually combined both. Called the 'father of modern surgery' and recognised as the greatest surgeon of the Renaissance, Paré introduced the modern treatment of wounds and amputations – ligature of arteries, popularised the truss for hernias, introduced artificial limbs and eyes and designed many new surgical instruments. He possessed all the qualities of a good surgeon: courage, ability, skilled hands and experience. Without academic qualifications, he learned his trade on the battlefield and became surgeon to four kings. Yet humility never left him and in his old age he could say of a patient: 'I dressed him and God healed him.' Nor did the drama of major surgery make him neglect other types of healing with his hands. He advocated the use of vigorous massage, and educated his students in the art of precise hand thrusts to align the vertebrae of the spine.

But the use of hands on the exterior of the body gradually fell into disuse. In more recent times the growing power of the medical profession weighed heavily on the lesser therapeutic arts. In Victorian England, both factors no doubt contributed to giving massage parlours the dubious reputation they retain today. On the continent, massage fared better. The Swedish fencing master Peter Henry Ling was acclaimed at least by the public for his successful exercise and massage techniques, and doctors in Germany and France as well as Scandinavia often practised the art 'without any thought of compromising their dignity', according to one commentator.

Throughout Europe these techniques flourished underground – a combination of folk medicine, bone-setting (not the term as we understand it today) and some of the old prescriptions of Hippocrates. The most common folk technique, practised from Spain to Russia, was back-walking; fraught with ritual, this simple method of massaging the spine with the feet was usually conducted by a woman, ideally the mother of twins or else a virgin. A British huntsman, Llewellyn Lloyd, described this scene which took place in a Swedish forest in the eighteenth century:

> Lumbago is cured by a woman that had twins trampling on the back of the sick man, who all the while lies with his face to the ground. While in this position he enquires several times of the woman, 'Why dost thou tramp on me?' to which she

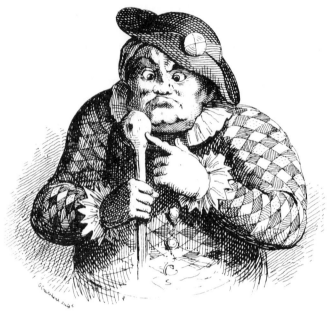

Sarah Mapp, bone-setter, caricatured by George Cruikshank

replies, 'Because I am better than thou art.' The patient then asks, 'Why art thou better than myself?' 'For the reason that I have borne under my breasts two hearts, two pair of lungs, two livers, four ears, four hands, and thou hast not.'

There are records of young girls being taught to stamp up and down on spines, of peasant women in Berwickshire relieving the back pains of others, of female camel drivers practising the art on one another in the Arabian desert. Pairs of people commonly manipulated each other's backs by interlocking arms back to back and alternately lifting each other – a technique called 'weighing salt'. In those days of heavy manual labour, back pains were so much a part of life that they were given names that translated as 'blood, or shot, of the witch'.

A more advanced form of manipulation for other parts of the body as well as the back was known as bone-setting. Likewise imbued with magical overtones, this technique was usually the special gift of a single farm family, and was passed down from one generation to the next. As in many forms of manipulation, the theory was simplistic: it was believed that pains were due to a small bone being out of place. Bone-setters were often skilled craftsmen and gained credibility by being able to set broken bones as well. When they acquired a reputation, they often made their way to the towns, there to join the quacks so despised by legitimate doctors. That they were ubiquitous throughout Europe is indicated by the names they acquired: *Kot-knackare* or 'spine knockers' in Scandinavia, *algebristas* in Spain, *renunctores* in Italy, *bailleuls* and *rebouteux* in France, and *Glieder-zetzen* in Germany.

Some bone-setters, such as Sarah Mapp, achieved notoriety. This eighteenth-century madcap, grotesquely caricatured by Cruik-shank and Hogarth, earned this famous description in the *London Magazine* of 2 August 1736:

> The Town has been surpriz'd lately with the Fame of a young woman at Epsom, who, tho' not very regular, it is said, in her Conduct has wrought such Cures that seem miraculous in the Bone-setting way. The Concourse of People to Epsom on this Occasion is incredible, and 'tis reckon'd she gets near to 20 Guineas a Day, she executing what she does in a very quick manner. . . . A Man came to her, sent, as 'tis supposed, by some Surgeons, on purpose to try her Skill, with his Hand bound up, and pretended his Wrist was put out, which upon Examination she found to be false, but to be even with him for his imposition, she gave him a Wrench, and really put it out, and bade him go to the Fools who sent him, and get it set again, or if he would come to her that Day a month, she would do it herself.
>
> This remarkable person is daughter to one Wallin, a Bone-setter of Hindon, Wilts. Upon some Family Quarrel she left her Father, calling herself Crazy Sally. Since she became famous, she married one Mr Hill Mapp, late Servant to a Mercer of Ludgate Hill, who, 'tis said, soon left her, and carried off £100 of her money.

Sarah went on to set up a practice in Pall Mall, catering to high society and even royalty and eventually being the subject of a play. Hounded by the surgeons of the day, one of whom characterised her as an 'ignorant, illiberal, drunken, female savage', she died a pauper.

To this day vestiges of the tradition of bone-setting can be observed throughout Europe. Pre-eminent among four famous prac-titioners in Ireland is an unpretentious farmer, Danny O'Neil, with whom I recently spent some time. With his sons he raises cattle and conducts a word-of-mouth clinic near Borris, in the southwest of Eire. A cynic might easily classify Danny's story as a case of blarney. Yet in this remote place he obviously gets both the simple and the most intractable cases – and he has visitors from throughout the British Isles.

Although people in the locality speak of a family tradition of bone-setting going back 800 years, he would not claim more than several generations, and in fact he grew up with no intention of pursuing his uncle's avocation – his father had ignored it. But shortly after the uncle died, he was approached by a man whose daughter had a badly dislocated wrist. 'You have the name, you have to be the one who does it,' he insisted. Reluctantly, Danny took the girl's wrist in his hand, even though he had never watched his uncle at work. As he described it to me, the feeling was miraculous: 'It was almost as if I could *see* what was wrong.'

Word spread, and soon Danny was repairing dislocations and broken bones that didn't require surgery. When he found he was able to correct a bad back that had confined a friend to his bed, he realised he had a power he should use. Today the mere mention of a bad back within 50 miles of his farm prompts the reply, 'Oh, you'll be wanting Danny O'Neil.' The road to his house has now been tarmacked, and a large car park, usually full throughout the day, greets the visitor; Danny has had to reserve a space for his own car.

His day of treatment begins at 8.30, just after milking. This is the first of three sessions, or surgeries, in the original sense of 'hand work'. But typically patients stream in and out without interruption, and Danny obliges them until the last one is gone in the evening. He takes a break from the consulting room occasionally to see another case in the yard: a cow with a bad back, a sheep with a dislocation, or a dog with a broken bone. They seem to suffer the same disasters that we do, and he treats them with the same matter-of-fact efficiency.

No doubt it is the speed and convenience of Danny's procedure that lures many of his patients – when the alternative is waiting for X-rays and going from one consultant to another. A bad-back case generally takes about five minutes. First Danny locates the point of trouble with his powerful fingers, and bends the patient forward and back as he continues to press on the centre of pain on the spine. Then the patient supports himself at arm's length from a wall. As Danny pushes strongly on the base of the spine with one hand, he lifts one leg straight out, usually bringing a gasp of surprise from his patient. He finishes his treatment by applying a wide strip of plaster across the point of trouble, to be left on for two weeks unless it becomes irritating. His standard advice is to sit upright in hard chairs rather than slouching in armchairs and to be careful about tripping or lifting heavy objects for several months. It all seems quite rational, even the poultice is made from a family recipe. And it does seem effective, since patients return years after their first treatment to correct the back they have thrown out again or for help with another problem. And then there are the rugby or hurling players, a demanding lot, who fill the parking spaces every Monday morning. . . .

The few Danny O'Neils in the world who still practise in an intuitive way, without training, must find it hard to resist the

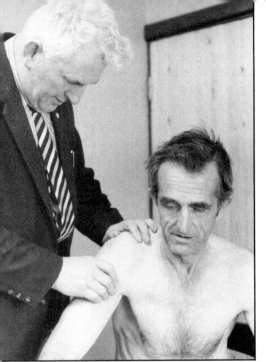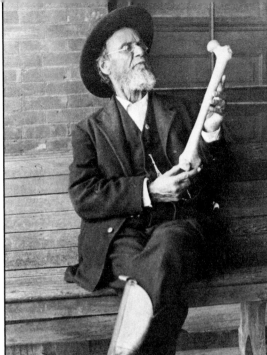

Left. Danny O'Neil, farmer and bone-setter, replacing a dislocated shoulder
Right. Andrew Taylor Still, 1828–1917, the founder of osteopathy

pressures of conformity. It's unlikely that Danny's sons will continue the tradition. Yet the fact remains that people are being helped in this minor but very human way: it is another face of medicine.

When a friend of Danny once tried to improve his work by bringing him books on anatomy and osteopathy, Danny found that they represented a barrier between the structure of the body and his instinctive sensitivity to it. Other practitioners approach the same body with a different vision: modern orthopaedic surgeons and physiotherapists, for example, for whom books and X-rays give the most revealing picture of this remarkable piece of natural machinery. These specialists nevertheless have much in common with the practitioners of folk medicine, with bone-setters, and with the long tradition of Hippocrates alluded to earlier. The use of traction, for example, in back cases was discussed thoroughly by Hippocrates, and commentaries on his works written in the tenth century included detailed drawings of the devices he had envisaged.

Finally, there are two nineteenth-century approaches to the structure of the body that form another link between ancient and modern 'hands on' medicine. The manipulative arts of osteopathy and chiropractic take the structure of the body as a starting point towards a general theory of illness and disease. Today these therapies are commonly considered to lie in the grey area of medical practice. The irony is that they were created in response to the reckless orthodox medicine of their day, a medicine that maimed and killed and had the audacity to call its competitors 'quacks'.

As will be seen in Chapter 5, on drugs, at the beginning of the nineteenth century doctors in Europe and even more so in America were practising what was perhaps the worst medicine in the world's history. Two men, both healers in pioneer farming communities in America, independently of each other began exploring alternatives to this lethal trade. Andrew Taylor Still and Daniel David Palmer both turned first to what was called 'magnetic' healing. Still was driven by tragic deaths in his family:

> War had left my family unharmed, but when the dark wings of spinal meningitis hovered over the land, it seemed to select my loved ones for its prey. . . . Day and night they nursed and cared for my sick and administered their most trustworthy remedies, but all to no purpose. . . . It was when I stood gazing upon three members of my family . . . all dead from the same disease, spinal meningitis, that I propounded to myself the serious question: in sickness had God left man in a state of guessing? . . . Like Colombus I trimmed my sail and launched my craft as an explorer.

Such extreme motivations are rare today in the protected world in which most of us live. It is a measure of Still's intensity that he devoted himself to magnetic therapy for several years before abandoning it. For a caring doctor, it was a seductive therapy. The word 'magnetic' came from its links with hypnosis, but it embodied everything we think of in a hands-on approach:

> By the friction of the hands along the spinal column, an invigorating life-giving influence is imparted to all the organs within the cavity of the trunk. The hand of kindness, of purity, of sympathy, applied here by friction combined with gentle pressure, is a singularly effective remedy for the morbid condition of the internal organs. It is a medicine that is always pleasant to take.

Thus one of its champions, Warren Felt Evans, contrasted it with the grotesque medicines of the day. The knowledge that spinal manipulation could affect diseases as well as aches and pains of the spine was not lost on Still as he travelled throughout the country practising a form of bone-setting. In his autobiography, published in 1908, he writes of the moment when he realised he was on the brink of a discovery:

> About 1880 . . . an Irish lady . . . had asthma in bad form, though she had only come to be treated for the pain in her shoulder. I found she had a section of upper vertebrae out of line, and I stopped the pain by adjusting the spine and a few ribs. In about a month she came back to see me without any pain or trace of asthma. . . .

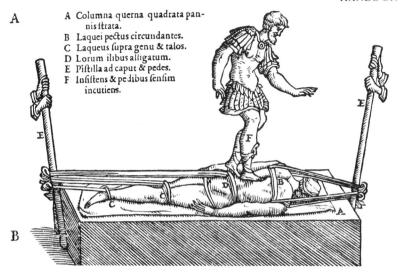

A Columna querna quadrata pan-
  nis ſtrata.
B Laquei peĉtus circundantes.
C Laqueus ſupra genu & talos.
D Lorum ilibus alligatum.
E Piſtilla ad caput & pedes.
F Inſiſtens & pedibus ſenſim
  incutiens.

These drawings of Hippocratic techniques for using traction and pressure to adjust vertebrae come from Galen's commentary on the ancient Greek doctor's writings. Similar techniques are still used by traditional practitioners in China

He speculated that there is a blocking of physical, not 'magnetic', fluids that causes disease, and that misplaced bones, especially those in the spinal column, are at fault. He had turned a folk medicine into a professional practice. Structure was to be the point of departure for the new healing art. Still dedicated his first book to 'the Master Architect and Builder'. This was the beginning of osteopathy.

A similar experience some fifteen years later convinced Palmer that adjusting spinal problems could have dramatic effects on seemingly unrelated illnesses. Anticipating the modern charge that 'anecdotal' evidence is not scientific, he later wrote the following about his first case, a long-standing one of deafness he cured with a sharp thrust to the patient's upper vertebrae:

> Knowledge of a single fact does not make a science . . . to know that a certain dorsal vertebra wrenched from its normal position was the cause of deafness; that the racking of it back into its former place would restore hearing; to know those two facts did not constitute a science; neither did it create the art of adjusting. But, so far it was specific knowledge and specific adjustment. It was the beginning of a science, not a new science, for the principles existed as far back as there were vertebrae.

In comparison with the other manipulative techniques discussed in this chapter, osteopathy and chiropractic are new and relatively untested fields. It is less than a hundred years since Palmer coined the term 'chiropractic' (hand practice) to describe his programme of

49

spinal alignment. Considering the scoffing and outright hostility his followers have endured, it is a tribute to the chiropractor's healing power that it has spread throughout the world. Osteopathy was equally damned by orthodox medicine, and Still used to challenge his patients with this proclamation:

> Remember that when many of you come to me you are not the most choice kind of patients. Remember the company you have kept before coming here. You have been with doctors who blister you, puke you, physic your toenails loose, fill your sides and limbs with truck from hypodermic syringes. You come to me with eyes big from Belladonna, backs and limbs stiff from plaster casts – you come with bodies suffering from all the diseases the flesh is heir to. Remember you have been treated and dismissed as incurable by all kinds of doctors before coming to us, and if we help you at all we do more than others have done.

In assembling a staff of practitioners for my clinic in Boston, the main resistance I have encountered between two disciplines has been the unwillingness of orthopaedic surgeons to work under the same roof as osteopaths or chiropractors. Tibetan healers have made rounds without animosity. Yet medical doctors argue that only a physician is entitled to prescribe a course of treatment, while manipulators of various kinds reject the idea of a doctor not qualified in their own speciality to say how a patient should be treated. Professional jealousy intensifies the conflict; osteopaths and chiropractors, though trained in a rigorous four-year programme, by their very

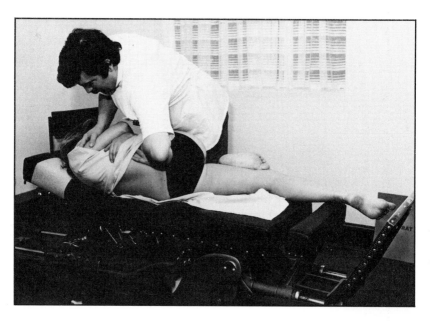

existence reproach doctors for failing to provide their patients with all the healing they require.

The argument is not all one-sided. The common complaint of doctors and medical societies is that chiropractors and osteopaths have in the past repeatedly made exaggerated, far-fetched claims. The spine is *not* the key that unlocks every illness, and claims of even partial success with many maladies show no discernible pattern – the hallmark of science. The manipulators answer that it is more important to get results than to construct an airtight theory.

The medical profession is aware of the financial as well as the professional challenge from these other men in white coats. The Victorian surgeon Sir James Paget stated the issue for his time: 'Few of you are likely to practise without having a bone-setter for a rival, and if he can cure a case you have failed to cure, his fortune will be made and yours marred.' In a leading article in 1871 about a famous bone-setter of the day, Richard Hutton, the *Lancet* went further in challenging the establishment:

> The late Mr Hutton . . . was for many years a sort of bugbear to not a few of the most distinguished surgeons of London; and every few months some fresh case was heard of in which he had given immediate and speedy cure to a patient who seemed vainly to have exhausted the legitimate skill of the metropolis. . . . It is quite manifest that quackery is only an expression of the extent to which legitimate practitioners fail to meet the desires of the sick. These desires may be

Left. Chiropractic. *Below*. Osteopathy: although there are differences between these two main systems of manipulation there are also similarities. The patient is usually placed in a position that allows a thrust or movement to have the desired effect

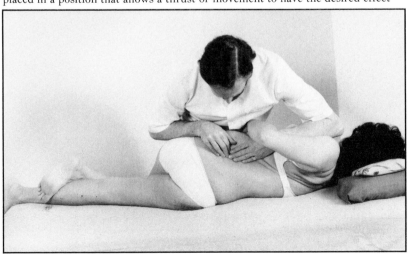

either reasonable or unreasonable, but they are sometimes perfectly reasonable; and then the medical practitioner who fails in fulfilling them, is the most effectual, indeed the only effectual, ally of the quack. If he does not know how to fulfill them, it is his duty to learn; and he in no way accomplishes this duty by railing at the quack for his failure or any mischief that he might do.

It is said that doctors gradually slipped away from the healing arts of the hand because they were regarded as manual labour, and dirty as well. Whatever the reasons in times past, these techniques are now missing from the curricula of medical schools. The treatment of back pain and other simple neuro-musculo-skeletal problems consists of pain-killers and rest. The loser is the patient who docilely heeds the warnings about these unscientific techniques. Then he is truly being manipulated.

Even though he is a paid professional a 'hands on' therapist appears to work on your body as an act of friendliness. It is like the attentiveness of a hospital visitor in India, who, instead of grapes or flowers, brings oil for a massage. As the fragrances fill the wards and deft hands work on bed-ridden bodies, one can sense a link being formed with the world outside. There are signs that this sort of personal contact is breaking down barriers of expected social conduct in the West. Athletes are no longer the sole users of exercise rooms, where massage has become a necessary adjunct to training. The benefits of massage for poor circulation, tissue swelling, frozen joints and muscular atrophy, adhesions and aches has become obvious. And massage just feels good. There are physiotherapy departments in many hospitals, where patients can attend classes not only to exercise unused muscles, but to learn how to reduce psychological tension through various forms of physical contact.

It is possible that the systems could co-operate. History has its examples. St Bartholomew's Hospital in London had a bone-setter on the staff in the 1600s and the Baghdad hospital of Avicenna in the eleventh century had manipulators. Very recently, a few hospitals in America and Britain have allowed chiropractors and osteopaths to work alongside conventional medical staff. Once the old prejudices have faded, an accommodation would mean an end to the railing and a beginning of mutual trust.

4 · NATURE'S · GREEN · PHARMACY

Try as we will to escape nature, it keeps pulling us back. We flee to the cities, we reject her food, and from nature's raw materials we distil exquisite poisons. Our modern pharmacopoeia is a jet-aircraft answer to illness, while nature lumbers along in a horse and cart. Herbs continue to fascinate man, however, as they have done since the dawn of history; yet there are as many aspects of herbs as there are of medicine itself. Let's look at three of them: my experience of a traditional Chinese pharmacy; the lessons of the long and intriguing story of herbalism; and a visit to herbalists practising in the west of England and in France.

Some of my most interesting training in China took place in that country's traditional pharmacies, whose stock in trade is based strongly, though not solely, on herbal remedies. Surrounded by a myriad plants, minerals and animal exotica among countless pills, lotions, liniments and powders, I felt like the sorcerer's apprentice.

Sometimes I would daydream about how the Cherokee Indians imagined the beginnings of plant medicine. It was animals, they said, that invented disease – to halt the spread of the human race. The plants found this out and summoned a council. Each plant agreed, when called upon by man in his distress, to furnish a remedy against the evil spell of the animals. Even the lowliest weed would offer its healing powers.

I sliced paper-thin layers of pilose deer antler, which the Chinese says quickens the dynamic forces of life; yes, I knew that according to scientific medicine the antler contains pantocine, which stimulates the adrenal gland. I ground the expensive inner bark of cinnamon, which 'moves and warms the energy'; in scientific language, it dilates the small capillaries. I dried tangerine peel, used to stimulate peristalsis in people with poor digestion. I broke buds off the twigs of ephedra, or woody horsetail, to concentrate its breath-restoring power for asthmatics. I boiled the fleece flower root in clay pots of

53

black bean soup to dampen its strong laxative properties; then it could be used safely for 'nourishing the essence that governs a graceful ageing process', or, as we say in the West, for lowering the blood cholesterol.

To impress our customers, we displayed the most expensive and rarest ingredients in full view, not unlike shopkeepers anywhere. Prominent in glass cases were the horns of Siberian antelope, which, when dispensed in powdered form, were useful in childhood fevers. Cows' gallstones, to be made into an antiseptic, nestled in elegantly carved miniature boxes. And the wild mountain ginseng, more precious than gold, rested in open chests of equal magnificence.

We stocked varying qualities and grades of each herb, in case the prescribing physician was fussy. Entire walls were covered with sealed boxes of pills, bottles and vials, each carefully labelled. The herbs were usually kept in drawers; the common ones were in jars on the counter, while sacks of dandelion-like herbs, the cheapest of all, remained in the back.

Like a medical brewery, this factory-storehouse-showroom teemed with unseen organic life. We had to be alert for mould, for infestation by insects, and for merchandise that had exceeded its shelf life. Now and then we whipped up special orders, grinding the ingredients into a fine powder, mixing in clarified honey as a preservative, rolling the whole thing into flat strips, snipping off pieces, then fashioning them into little balls.

My most pleasurable task was filling prescriptions. Unlike the ballpoint scribbles doctors dash off in the West, these orders were often executed with flowing, calligraphic brush strokes. The recipes – for that's what they were in most cases – might contain five or as many as twenty ingredients, but all were inscribed in large, exaggerated Chinese characters to obviate errors of eyesight. Patients asked me questions as I filled their orders – gathering the ingredients, weighing them on an old Chinese scale, mixing and wrapping. I began to feel like more than a pharmacist: I was a transmitter of nature's secrets to my fellow men. At the time I could not know that, along with learning the craft of the Chinese pharmacy, I was playing a small part in the herbal revivial that was taking place worldwide.

Now, many years after my training at the pharmacy, instead of working at my hospital clinic I return one day each week to being a herbalist. No longer the apprentice, I'm the sorcerer himself. Yet I don't think of herbs as competing with prescription drugs, nor do I fall into the trap of valuing herbs because they somehow mimic or provide the essential ingredient in drugs. In fact, when I encounter a true believer in herbalism I use my authority, when necessary, to convince the patient of the value of an antibiotic or a beta-blocker or simple aspirin. I recognise the value of lithium for manic depression, and birth control pills as part of a lifestyle choice. For most of my patients, however, any such advice is pointless.

Who are my patients? Most have already been to Boston's prestigious hospitals and clinics. They are chronically ill and desperate. Something has gone wrong with their stomachs, livers, lungs or reproductive organs. Their skin is blemished or ashen. They have fears that make no sense, memories that do not work, tumours that must come out. For one reason or another their cases are so severe or so complex that they have not been helped by the scientific healers. Typically they have tried so many drugs that they are themselves amateur prescribers, and they are exhausted from their unwanted education.

I listen to what they say about themselves and their fantasies. Then I select a combination of herbs that matches the pattern of illness – and health – that I see in each patient. Finding a herb that relieves a particular symptom is one consideration, but my main task is to sense the dominant texture, quality, or 'rhythm' of each person's being. Is it like the crackling moments in a blazing fire, to use a Chinese metaphor? Or, to use a Greek picture of illness, is it like a melancholic, overcast autumn day? Or a simpler image – a vibrant spring afternoon? Then I add enough of the right combination of herbs to fit the person, to help any changes take hold and grow.

Herbs have pharmacological activating principles which can be determined in a laboratory, but to some people, including myself, it sometimes seems they also have many 'souls'. Milk vetch, for example, stimulates the central nervous system, increases urination, lowers blood pressure and inhibits the growth of various microorganisms; this is its scientific essence. But untrained peasants also know that this common weed has a quaint, folksy spirit, and when a relative or neighbour doesn't seem quite well they tell him or her, 'Milk vetch is good for tiredness.' And I know it also has a magical 'soul'. This long black root with a bright yellow centre exudes the persuasive power of transformation, the power to change darkness into light. Finally this herb, like all the rest, has its artistic soul with its own texture and pulse, a way of interacting with other herbs and indeed with bodily sensations and feelings not measurable in the biochemist's lenses and scales. The 'soul' of each herb may be known to the journeyman herbalist, but the feeling for their mixture, balance and synergetic effects constitutes the art of herbalist medicine. In contrast, science proceeds by isolating active ingredients of natural substances, reducing everything as far as laboratory equipment will permit – and then warning patients not to combine particular medications with others.

Milk vetch is rarely used alone. Scientific descriptions are inadequate to describe its action: it acts like a catalyst in that it is an activator, but it also contributes something of itself to the ultimate reaction. When combined with ginger, it stimulates digestion; with plantain seeds, it assuages chronic oedema; with ephedra twigs, it promotes sweating, whereas with ephedra root it inhibits sweating; with eucommia bark, it helps lower blood pressure, while with ginseng it raises blood pressure.

So far, we have only dipped our toes into the science versus herbalism issue. Now it is time to go beyond poetic terms and to look a little further. Because herbalism, unlike science, is not analytically based that does not mean it's irrational. To a herbalist healer, it might seem irrational to extract a chemical from a plant and throw the rest away; yet this is how pharmaceutical companies proceed. Chemicals derived from ergot, rauwolfia or foxglove form important components of modern medicine. No doubt the search for new drugs will continue among plants, bushes and trees, but this will not result in new faith in herbalism. Whatever chemists discover will only superficially affect their opinion of herbs.

The new breed of herbalist, armed with the tools of the chemist in addition to those of tradition and folklore, insists that the value of his therapeutic is greater than the value of all the chemicals that can be extracted from all the herbs. His reasoning goes like this. The isolation of a chemical sharpens its cutting edge, so to speak: in life-or-death situations or when dealing with severe problems, precision, quick absorbency and extreme potency are valuable. In chemotherapy, for example, laboratory-like precision is often called for. But herbs have different advantages – not because of some vague concept of 'naturalness', but because of several observable qualities that result from *not* being broken down into single identifiable chemicals.

First, a whole herb is rarely fast-acting or extremely potent; in many chronic conditions a slow approach is desirable. Certainly there are abundant poisons in nature, and strong herbs can have side effects. It's not that herbs are necessarily without danger but that they're usually clinically gentler. Crude preparations of herbs taken by mouth release active ingredients into the bloodstream relatively slowly. Their concentrations are low and other inert compounds slow absorption.

Second, the biochemical effect of a plant depends on the totality of the organic and inorganic substances in it. The same active ingredient within a plant has remarkably different effects when it is isolated from the plant. It almost seems as if there is a balancing mechanism in the naturally occurring substances of a plant which prevent it going out of control. Consider these examples.

Of the twenty-two different drugs in opium that we know of, including codeine and papaverine, the active ingredient or dominant one is morphine. But morphine and opium affect the same person quite differently. The synergy among morphine and the other drugs changes its effects. Foxglove contains digitalis, one of the most important heart medications. But because foxglove also contains verodoxin, a supposedly inert substance, a lower dosage of the intact plant form achieves the same results as a higher dose of the extract. Both are toxic, but the initial side effect of the plant is only nausea, whereas the drug produces heart arrhythmia. The dandelion plant is an important diuretic, strangely blessed with about three times the potassium content of an ordinary green-leaved plant. Most chemical diuretics unfortunately leach potassium from the body. The herb ephedra's active ingredient is the alkaloid ephedrine, commonly used to treat asthma. The crude plant contains other alkaloids (such as pseudoephedrine) that counter the side effects of ephedrine, such as increased blood pressure and heart rate. This can confer a considerable therapeutic advantage on a patient.

Third, the complexity of the alkaloids in any plant leads to effects that cannot be explained by the on-off mechanism of an isolated drug. For example, the dosage of herb can be so critical as to reverse its effects; schisandra fruit in one dosage stimulates the central nervous system and in another dampens it. In the presence of various other herbs, notoginseng reduces the clotting time of blood; in other circumstances it can promote circulation and dilate such vessels as the coronary artery. The action of Chinese angelica root on the uterus is unexplainable by the one-drug, one-effect theory; it can both relax a tight uterus and contract a loose one. This regulating effect is even more prominent in herbal combinations. For example, there is a famous twelfth-century Chinese recipe of six herbs called the Six-flavour Rhemannia pill: it can lower the blood pressure of an agitated person, known to Western doctors as a 'Type A' individual, and raise the pressure of the same type patient with low blood pressure. The active ingredients of this mixture have been isolated in the laboratory: there are more than 100 and they have no effect on hypertension! Their combined effect, rather, is on the Type A personality.

It may never be possible for the new herbalist to prove his case on the scientist's own terms, for science has the admirable virtue of being able to adjust to each new piece of evidence with yet another adjustment in its theoretical structure. Reduction is its strength and its weakness – weakness because in pursuing its ideal of isolation it sometimes can move only further and further from the whole.

The medical soup kitchen of herbalism seems to have been bubbling for at least 60,000 years. Archaeologists dug up more than bones in their recent excavation of a Neanderthal burial site in what is now northern Iraq. Higher levels of pollen from eight plant species turned up in soil analysis, and seven of those eight are still used by the herbalists of this region – in fact, worldwide. Someone put them there, for a reason we can only guess at. Someone roamed the nearby hills gathering the tiny, daisy-like yarrow, effective against dysentery and intestinal colic; blue bonnet, a valuable diuretic and astringent, and a useful eyewash; and ephedra, helpful in asthma and also in fever and arthritis.

I am a herbalist rather than a botanist; in the field I'm not sure if I could tell the most common herb from the next. But I find everything about herbs fascinating reading, including their association with food, their long history in every culture, and their comparison with modern drugs.

Our hunter-gatherer ancestors seem to have thoroughly explored their flora and fauna. To the 700 known edibles of prehistoric times, not one natural foodstuff has been added to this day. The poisons were carefully weeded out – curare, ovabain, veratrin, boundou – and some were tamed. The milky juice of the *Manihot* plant contains deadly hydrocyanic acid: early man washed this out of the plant which was then heated to yield the highly nutritious tapioca. Between the poisons and the foods were the herbs, but the boundaries were as indistinct then as now. Foods like fruit can act as laxatives; herbs like aconite (monkshood), which can strengthen a weak heart, can easily be toxic. In the earliest Chinese medical

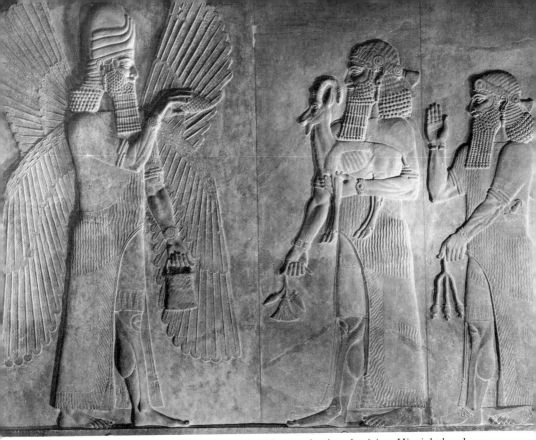

On the right of this eighth-century BC Assyrian carving is a physician. His right hand is in a position of prayer while his left holds a three-headed poppy plant, the source of pain-relieving opium

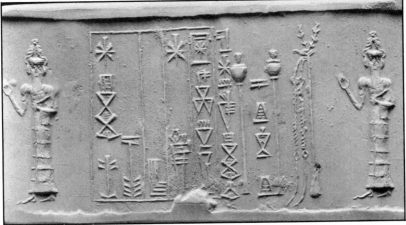

An impression in clay of a doctor's seal, the oldest known medical card. Dr Urlugale-dina was a Babylonian, practising about 4000 years ago. The card shows that he used the three branches of Babylonian medicine: *left*, divine intervention – the God holding a remedy; *centre*, surgery – some knives; *right*, herbs – the pestle and mortar used for crushing them

writings, all medicines are referred to as poisons. American Indians called them 'powers'. Galen tried to settle the issue in the second century by saying that the body 'overcomes' food but that medicines are 'victorious' over the body.

Studies of present-day tribes indicate that from the beginning primitive people turned to herbs in time of sickness. Bowel evacuation, vomiting, sweating, urination, inflammation, coughs, insomnia, parasites, menstruation and various injuries and pain were all dealt with by the application of specific herbs. I have mentioned only a fragment of the numerous herbs whose effects can be explained by their chemical properties: the correlation is extremely close. Herbs obviously worked.

The first important record of herbs, from the Egyptian Ebers Smith Papyrus, a copy of writings going back some twenty-five centuries BC, lists 876 prescriptions and some 500 substances. Some, such as frankincense, senna, juniper berries and aloe are well known; some, for instance opium, castor oil and gentian, are still used today in chemical derivatives. Some seem logical (liver for night blindness), others fanciful (rattlesnake fat for baldness, the faeces of horseflies for a baby's tantrums). The minerals would be included in a nutrition manual even today: iron, lead, magnesium, lime and soda. Like physicians everywhere, this Egyptian expected his prescriptions to be followed precisely. The plant or animal was described carefully and the dosage, application and time of day laid down.

Ancient Babylonian clay tablets, unearthed in what was an ancient pharmacy, show an equally sophisticated apothecary. Among the 230 medicines on the shelves were drugs that would impress a London chemist: myrrh, an anti-microbial and anti-inflammatory; mandrake, containing the familiar narcotic scopolamine; and belladonna, containing what is still one of scientific medicine's best anti-spasmodics, atropine.

The chemical properties of herbs were unknown to the herbalists of Egypt and Babylon. For them the soul of their craft was magic, pure and simple. Trial and error, observation and conjecture convinced them of the efficacy of their compounds, but they attributed this to the steady hand of the gods – that is, demons of all sorts. In prescribing for a toothache, a Babylonian druggist would undoubtedly include some henbane, a potent narcotic poultice, but he would also insist that it was applied while facing west, and that the sufferer should shun moonlight, avoid eating eels, and chant this charm with each application:

The evil ones of Ea
They stand on the highway to befoul the path;
Evil are they, seven are they –
By heaven be ye exorcised! By Earth be ye exorcised!
O worm, may Ea break thee with this powerful hand.

The herb was considered animate, something that could be coerced to work by the god of wisdom, Ea. It was thought to work, in what we would consider a simple logical fallacy, by means of a resemblance with its purpose. The lungs of the fox, a long-winded animal, were used in chronic respiratory problems, for instance. There was also the idea that every living thing affected and resonated with everything else, including the spirits and demons; resemblance was supposed to help the resonance.

If it's hard to stomach the logic of prescribing yellow herbs for jaundice, red herbs for blood problems, and cashew nuts for kidneys, when we come to the Chinese the puzzle intensifies. In my classes in pharmacognosy – the study of the drug properties of crude natural substances – in China I came across many herbs that were historically rationalised by the process of resemblance. The Chinese herbalist treats night blindness, for example, with bat faeces! My modern Chinese textbook kept saying that such therapies pass scientific tests, but few results are available in Western languages. Well, bat faeces are full of undigested mosquito eyes and bats fly in the dark . . . magical reasoning, yes. But this excreta is also rich in vitamin A! Maybe that's why the Chinese don't use owl faeces.

Perhaps a joint commission of sorcerers and scientists should be convened to set the boundaries. I say this not frivolously, but after learning that the faeces of the flying squirrel, prescribed for intestinal distension, has been shown in the laboratory to relax spasms of smooth muscle. And that sloughed snake skin, a natural candidate for skin problems, actually has anti-histamine properties. And that decoctions from rhinoceros horn really do strengthen the hearts of dogs, cats and frogs. The commission must open with a chant!

I am always brought back to earth by the Greeks. They are responsible for the Western herbalism we know today, free of the magical shroud, grounded in observation of results, yet still closely related to interpretation of the unified person, the patient and not the disease. The Hippocratic writings in their completeness mention in passing 250 medical plants, without incantations. A pupil of Aristotle later compiled the first book in history, Eastern or Western, devoted to the powers of individual herbs – the *Rhizotomikon*.

Finally, in the late first century a Greek doctor in the army of Nero's Rome produced the *magnum opus* of herbalism. Dioscorides summarised the state of the art to his day, covering some 600 plants and 350 animal and mineral substances. His *Peri Hulas Iatrikos*, or *About Medical Trees*, came to be known in Latin by the confident title *De Materia Medica*. With a large drawing of each entry, a description of appearance, medical qualities and preparation, and warnings of side effects, it is the prototypical herbal.

In the second century AD appeared Galen, physician to Marcus Aurelius, author of more than a hundred medical texts, and one of the greatest herbalists then and perhaps ever. He codified the Graeco-Roman medical system, including thirty books on remedies. Not only did he systematically record herbal effects on each sensation, but he quantified them too. His degrees of effectiveness ranged from 'unnoticed' to 'openly', 'intensely' and 'completely'. For example, he listed anise and garlic as 'warm and dry to the third degree'. This system of classification was the bible of the Western herbalist for 1500 years.

Independently of the West, it would seem, the

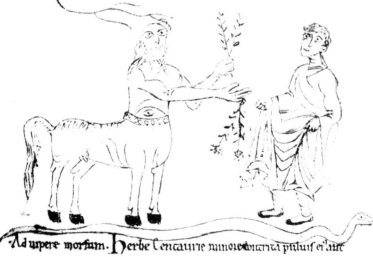

This page from a twelfth-century Anglo-Saxon herbal shows a mingling of ideas from different cultures. In Greek legend the centaur, Chiron, discovered the healing powers of herbs. Here he is giving a herb to a physician while at their feet the Teutonic worm of disease flees from the magic in the herb

Chinese codified their system at about the same time. The *Divine Husbandman's Materia Medica* lists 365 remedies in much the same way as Dioscorides put them down. The two traditions followed a similar path some 1500 years later, when the most famous Chinese herbal, Li Shi-zhen's *Great Materia Medica*, appeared in 1578, only fifty-eight years before the massive work of John Parkinson. There were 1892 medicines in the Chinese work, 3800 in the London herbal. The latter was influenced heavily by the Moslem tradition, which, as we have seen, made a strong impact on European scholarship. In the thirteenth century Ibn Baitar's *Jami* was the principal storehouse of their herbal knowledge, with some 2000 entries. India's books are difficult to date, but it seems clear that their medical tradition dates back as far as the Greek and Chinese philosophical eras and their earliest texts mention 600 herbs. Only recently has any progress been made in exploring the roots of American Indian and African herbalism. The Aztecs had some 1200 herbs. Zulu herbalists use up to 200 herbs and know of over 700 herbs.

A Buddhist legend captures the universal appeal of herbalist thought. For the final examination of medical students, a teacher leads them to the forest; he asks them to disperse and bring back as many plants as they can which are of no medical value. After two or three days most of the students have returned, each with a few plants. On the fifth day, the last student appears empty-handed and sad. 'You,' says the teacher, 'are the only one qualified to pursue the herbal path.'

At the high point of Western herbalism in the seventeenth century John Gerard, herbalist to James I, grew more than a thousand varieties in his London garden. Others he collected from the marshes around what is now Paddington Station, or in the ditches around Piccadilly Circus. This curious item of information was relayed to me by Michael McIntyre, who conducts a phone-in programme on herbalism on Radio Oxford, and with his wife Ann practises herbal medicine at their home in the Cotswolds.

Because of my academic excursions into Chinese herbalism, with some Arabic, Greek and native American influence, I was anxious to see another sort of practitioner in the McIntyres. The garden at their stone cottage in the countryside was full of tall lupins, mallows, angelica, foxgloves, hollyhocks and marigolds, and I was immediately enveloped by the scent of mint, marjoram, rosemary, thyme, lavender, sage, balm and basil. Ann told me their patients' healing process always began here, before they ever reached the clinic. I was slightly embarrassed by the fact that my book-learning had not prepared me to recognise some of my close friends in their natural habitats.

Their clinic had the crisp look of any good medical practice. Inside I faced my second surprise: a full wall of shelves containing tiny, smoke-dark bottles. They contained tinctures, extracts of medical plants in water or alcohol, and they had been made by the McIntyres under special government licence. They had previously gathered most of the herbs themselves. Even the dried herbs, in large jars bearing neatly printed labels in Latin, came from nearby fields or had been sought out on special expeditions to Ireland, Corfu, Italy, France and the mountains of Switzerland.

The McIntyres collect their own herbs because it is a guarantee of quality. Fortunately, they live some distance from the lead-laden atmosphere of busy roads and from most agricultural spraying. Yet it is still a tricky business, only possible from late spring to the first frost of winter, and always threatened by environmental pollution.

Michael and Ann met as one of the side effects, as he explains it, of herbal medicine. They were both students at the 120-year-old National Institute of Medical Herbalists; the four-year course was every bit as demanding as that for his degree in history at Oxford, Michael told me. He had also worked as an editor in a London publishing house which is where he first came across herbalism in a book on alternative medicines. He was hooked. Ann's journey was more circuitous: she had taken part in a programme of aid to Indian tribes in a remote jungle area of Colombia. Inspired by their success with the curious power of herbs, she decided to explore this answer to the dangers and short supply of drugs.

Michael's first afternoon patient was a new one, and not untypical of those who come to the practice. His colitis had reached the stage at which drugs were losing their effect, and his specialist had advised intestinal surgery to relieve the pain and diarrhoea. Herbs had been suggested as a last resort, and after an examination Michael agreed that the situation, even though advanced, was far from hopeless. The consultation took about an hour, at the end of which a logical prescription emerged. It consisted of single tincture, to be taken four times a day, combining a number of cooling and calming herbs: goldenseal to relieve the inflammation of the gut, marshmallow and comfrey to soothe the irritated organs, agrimony and shepherd's purse to help astringe the damaged tissue and stop the diarrhoea, wild Mexican yam and chamomile for relief against spasms and pain,

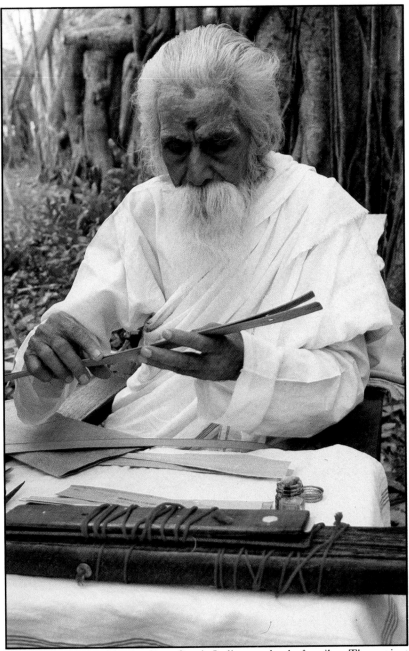

Shri Ramachandra Sharma from South India, a palm leaf scribe. The ancient Indian texts have always been written down on palm leaves, but these suffer from insects and wear. During the last 2000 years scribes have often made new copies of the Ayurvedic medical writings

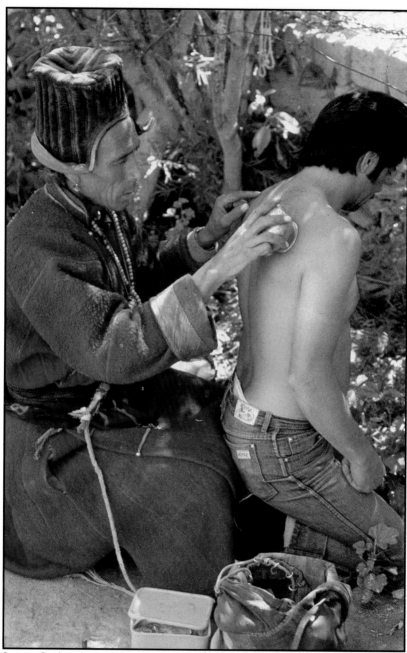

Sonam Gyelson is a country doctor practising Tibetan medicine in Ladakh. Tibetan medicine began with a conference held in the seventh century AD. Physicians trained in Greek, Indian and Chinese medicine collaborated to create a synthesis of their knowledge, with elements of tribal medical knowledge and Buddhism

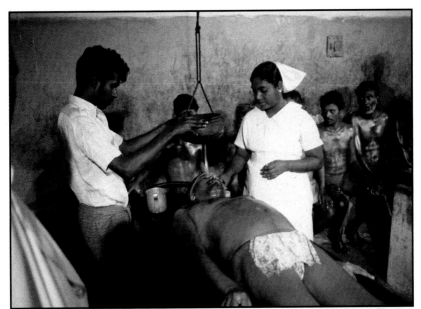

These massages, called panchakarma, have a powerful effect on patients. To prevent them from becoming too hot they are cooled by a stream of coconut milk which is poured on to their foreheads

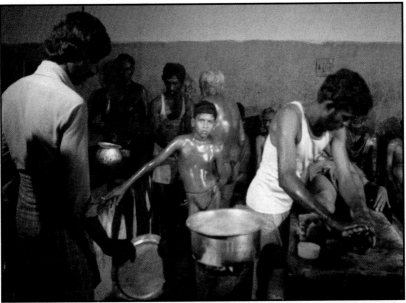

Ayurvedic medicine relies heavily on massaging complex mixtures of herbs into the skin, through which they pass into the system. The massage room of the Arignar Anna Hospital in Madras is busy all day with patients suffering from a wide range of conditions; some seemingly intractable ones appear to be relieved

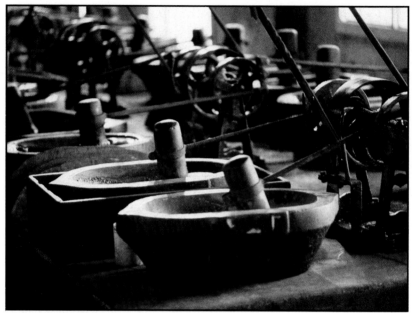

The preparation of Ayurvedic medicines is big business in India. These mechanised pestles and mortars match the grinding action of the hands that traditionally prepared the ingredients. They are at work in the factory of the Indian Medical Practitioners' Co-operative Society, Madras

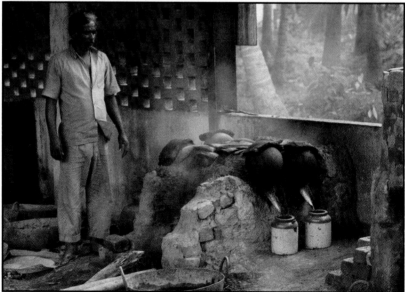

Although the Co-operative Society makes large quantities of both patent medicines and drugs for doctors to prescribe, its techniques of distillation are still those which were once employed by the alchemist

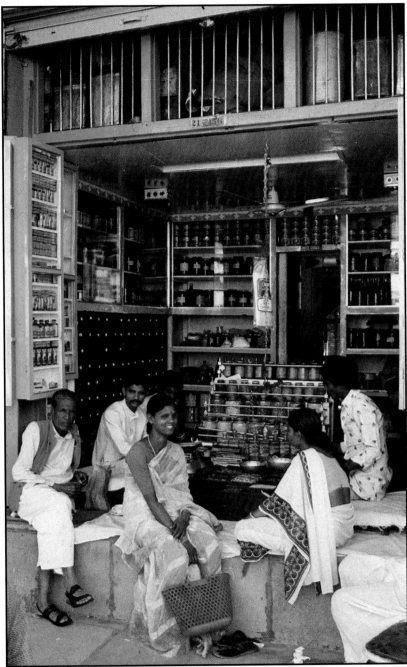

A Unani pharmacy in the city of Hyderabad, the main centre for ancient Greek medicine in India. The medicine of Hippocrates is still practised in India today. This pharmacy also acts as an informal meeting place

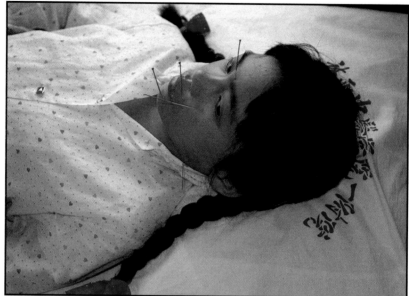

The Chinese have a practical, unromantic attitude to acupuncture; for them there is nothing exotic about it. When they become ill they decide whether to go to the 'Western' clinic, or to the traditional Chinese one where they choose a herbal doctor or acupuncture. They have a clear idea of the relative merits of the various systems; usually choosing science for urgent conditions and tradition for long-term problems

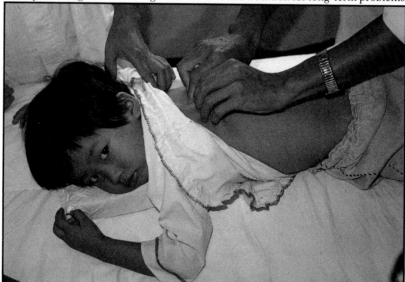

Acupuncture in China is practised regularly on young children. They sometimes cry when the needle is first inserted but usually they become quiet and relaxed for the rest of the treatment time. Acupuncture is used primarily for healing purposes rather than as an anaesthetic

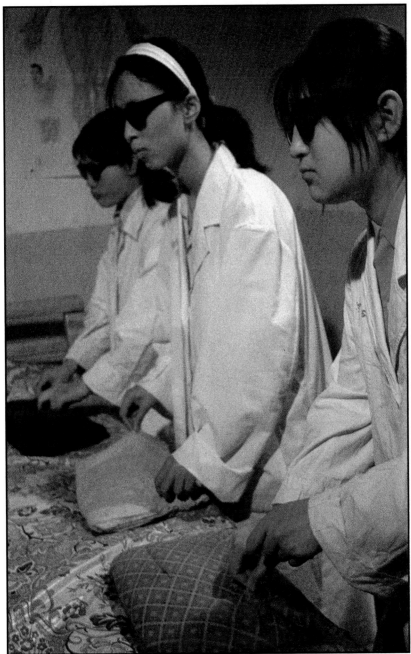

Blind girls at the school for massage in Chengdu practise one of the twenty finger-strengthening exercises that they do every day. Massage and manipulation has always been a way of life for blind people in China, partly because it protects the modesty of patients

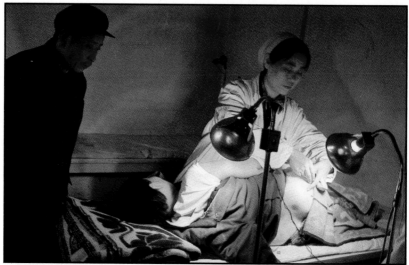

Using acupuncture in the winter in parts of China may sometimes cause problems for those hospitals that lie below the 'Heating Line', where buildings are not heated. In these circumstances, only essential parts of the skin are bared, and the patient is often kept warm by radiant electric lights

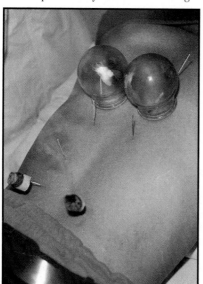

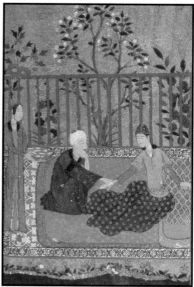

Left. Here the doctors are using the three main techniques of the acupuncturist: they have placed needles in some points; on top of two of these they have placed cylinders of burning herbs; and they are cupping, which has a strong local effect on blood supply and the surrounding tissue

Right. The qualities of the pulse inform the doctor of the internal texture of the balance of a patient. Here a fifteenth-century Moslem doctor takes his patient's pulse

and cowslip and lemon balm to reduce the mental distress all too evident in the interview. Without a dietary upheaval – throwing out all fried and processed foods and coffee – Michael warned that there was little chance for the herbs to work. After all, they only 'nudge' the body; they do not attack it. With a few words about a breathing exercise for relaxation, Michael sent his patient on his way. The next appointment was not arranged for next week, or two weeks hence, but for next month. I learned later that no operation had been needed.

The unspoken rule of medicine is diagnose, diagnose, diagnose. I next visited a typical practice in Paris, the clinic of Dr Paul Balaiche, to witness another diagnosis. Dr Balaiche, like all French herbalists a medical doctor, holds the newly created chair of herbalism at the University of Paris Nord.

The examination I was privileged to observe proceeded differently from the one in the west of England, in a highly charged scientific ambience. In France, the scientific medical profession leads the movement. Herbs are produced by large companies for use by thousands of doctors. The middle-aged woman in the examining room had come here after years of conventional treatment which had failed to relieve her urinary infection. Antibiotics, the surgical stretching of her urethra, and finally psychiatric help had all failed. Dr Balaiche took a urine sample and asked the patient to return the next day. Meanwhile he tested the essential oils of seventy plants on cultures of the urine. The next day he prescribed various herbal oils containing anti-bacterial, anti-spasmodic, diuretic and carminative properties; they were the oils that had reacted positively on the plates of urine cultures. He prescribed with confidence. Dr Balaiche has achieved a success rate of better than 80 per cent with herbal treatment of several thousand women suffering from cystisis which had failed to respond to conventional treatment. He has also performed successful double-blind tests. This is one of the factors that prompted the French medical establishment to recognise *phyto-thérapie*, as it is called in France, as part of the orthodox tradition.

I have come a long way from my student days in the Chinese pharmacy. I have seen the world change from the time when I was looked on with suspicion, because I was the first and for a while the only Westerner in my Third World school, to now, only a dozen years later, when one of the finest medical schools in France is reaching out to nature's green pharmacy. The medicinal herbs are like weeds: sometimes rejected, sometimes tolerated, and sometimes rediscovered and prized anew. Their strengths and weaknesses are different from cultivated plants and it is unlikely they will disappear.

5 · ENTER · MAGIC · BULLETS

If our élite drug companies were to trace their lineage, they might blush to discover that the guiding principle of what they do was the inspired idea of a sixteenth-century doctor who has variously been described as a mountebank, a visionary and a drunken fool. His very name conjures mystery and unreality: Paracelsus, which he dubbed himself in honour of the Roman Celsus, author of the first medical text to be printed.

The printing press itself might be credited with launching the modern era of medicine. The wide distribution of books after the middle of the fifteenth century did generate an explosion of new ideas. Paracelsus himself was the first to write a medical text in the vernacular, to bring new medical thinking to the common people. And it was to ordinary people that Paracelsus appealed and ministered, much like the religious reformers of his day. Indeed, Paracelsus came to be known as the Martin Luther of medicine, so revolutionary was his insistence on experience as the basis of medical science, and so devoted was he to the poor. And yet, though he can rightly be called the first environmentalist, the father of chemotherapy, and the inspiration of homeopathy, he was sadly ahead of his time. Today his many books are dismissed as the ravings of a madman, and he is politely ignored. But history is full of examples of mankind's short memory. Aristotle's biology, recognised as the basis of modern science, was forgotten for twelve centuries; and in our own day physicists look the other way when confronted with Heisenberg's metaphysical speculations. The colourful life of Paracelsus, born about 1493, forms an appropriate introduction to the story of modern drugs.

He was born Aureolus Theophrastus Bombastus von Hohenheim in a Swiss mining town where his father was a doctor and a teacher of metallurgy. The young Paracelsus toiled in the mercury mines and smelters before entering medical school, and it was this experience with metals that gave rise to the 'different line of thought', to use Heisenberg's phrase, that was destined to bring chemistry to the service of medicine.

After a few years of conventional medical practice and a period spent teaching at the University at Basle, he overturned all the tables of his profession, announcing that he had 'found the medicine which I had learned was faulty, and that those who had written about it neither knew nor understood it. . . . I had to look for another approach.' It is not surprising that, after burning the texts of Galen and Avicenna in a public bonfire, 'so that all this misery should go up in the air in smoke', he was asked to find other employment. For the next dozen years of his short life he wandered throughout Europe, from Spain and Holland to Turkey and Russia, pursuing the secrets of nature.

A measure of his genius is that in this short period he became the most famous practitioner in Europe. Among his patients were the most learned man of his time, Erasmus; the richest, Fugger, who gave birth to the munitions industry; and the great printer and publisher, Frobenius. Everything about Paracelsus seemed extreme. He liked silk garments, but wore them until they fell off in rags. He sought out the poorest for treatment, and sided with them in the peasant wars that raged throughout central Europe. He advanced his thought by quarrelling, accurately assessing himself: 'I pleased no one except the sick whom I cured.'

Like many other scientists whom we revere for their supposedly serene rationality – Kepler and Newton come to mind – Paracelsus indulged in the grey area of speculation characteristic of the times: astrology, alchemy and magic. There was no limit to his energy for enquiry; he expected to find the key to the healing of man in man himself, consulting 'old women, gypsies, magicians, wayfarers, and all manner of peasant folk and random people'. A devout Christian, he believed that within man there burned a primal spiritual urge, to be tapped in faith healing, in prayer and in the 'power of the word', that simply by describing illness or death, healing and the relief of pain could be induced. It was in chemistry, however, that he touched the nerve that would resonate to our own times. The true art of prescribing medicine, he concluded, 'consists in extracting . . . in the discovery of that which is concealed in things'. It may have seemed to him to be 'the concealed finger of God', but he sought it in the chemistry of metals and the distillations of poisons borrowed from the Arabs and the herbalists. With fire he purified such minerals as arsenic, sulphur, lead, copper, iron, silver and mercury to release their 'arcanum', or specific virtue. With his daring insight he took preparations of the older medicines, often poisonous and reserved for external application, and refined them into palatable doses. One of his favourites was antimony, a powerful irritant that can cause heart failure. He lined cups with antimony so that it would seep into wine, creating a purge to bring on vomiting or heavy sweating. The ancients limited mercury to external use, since it can cause tremors, frightening grimaces, loss of teeth and even death. Paracelsus worked it into a salt solution in tiny amounts, and used it as a diuretic for oedema. He was inevitably accused of poisoning his patients. 'All things are poison,' he replied, 'it is the dosage that makes a thing not a poison.' We are reminded of the chemicals in table salt, and of the current debate over artificial sweeteners as possible carcinogens.

It was a logical step from the development of these 'magic bullets' to the concept of highly specified diseases. Though we take this concept for granted today, in his era disease was still perceived according to the ancient model of disharmony of natural forces throughout the person. Paracelsus was one of the first to explain diseases as 'things' that possessed specific traits regardless of the constitution of the patient; anticipating germ theory, his followers called them 'thorns that had to be removed'. The Black Death from the Old World and new plagues believed to come from the New World, such as syphilis, made identifiable imprints on old and young, sanguine and phlegmatic alike. This was no mere theoretical exercise: Paracelsus was the first to identify and treat a hazard of the working environment, a lung disease of miners. The old medicine, from 'the balanced way' to herbalism, thought in terms of humoral illness and was too slow to react to new diseases; the new medicine thought in terms of specific disease and could react rapidly.

When this scruffy, belligerent, wild-eyed, paradoxical prophet died as the result of a tavern brawl, he left behind him a movement that would soon overpower the green pharmacy. This subversion was aided by a small fifth column of drug-like herbs that came from the New World, introduced for specific diseases: Peruvian bark, or quinine, for malaria; ipecac for dysentery; guiac and sarsaparilla for syphilis; and cocaine for pain. Entrepreneurs joined forces with fashionable doctors in a parallel to modern medico-industrial complexes. Laudanum and mercury-chloride, concoctions of Paracelsus himself, would remain the reigning drugs of choice for three centuries.

Like any other human activity, medicine has a way of overdoing a good thing. Enthusiasm for initial success leads to excess. But chemical medicine proved to be a particularly bad offender; herbalism was being driven from the field. If herbs were adopted, it was to be on a new basis. In 1785 William Withering of Edinburgh published his findings on digitalis, or foxglove, still one of our most consistent heart medications, and laid down this challenge: '. . . rejecting the fables of the ancient herbalists, build only upon the basis of accurate and well-conceived experimentation'. It didn't matter that he had taken the drug from the herbalist's own armoury, from 'an old woman in Shropshire who had sometimes made cures after the more regular practitioners had failed'. Experimentation was being carried to deplorable extremes by anyone with access to highly toxic substances: arsenic, antimony, strychnine, tartar emetic and the doctors' favourite, calomel – mercury-chloride.

The symptoms of treatment by calomel were appalling. 'Within a few days after ingestion, severe stomatis with excessive salivation appeared. Patients had ulcerated lips, cheeks, and tongue, soreness and inflammation of the gums, plus loosening and frequent loss of teeth,' a recent history of American medical practices reads. Children were frequent victims of fused or knotted jaws, with resulting gangrene and osteomyelitis. Cramps and diarrhoea were common, but were typically attributed to the disease. Larger doses were said to produce a sedative effect, no doubt as a side effect of mercury poisoning. Combined with the prevalent practice of bleeding, calomel made the 'heroic' efforts of doctors a grim travesty. George Washington was treated for a sore throat with 14 grams of calomel and relentless bleeding, which killed him. Calomel was so common that a German anatomist of the times wrote that mercury was a constituent of bones – because he saw it in all of his assays.

We have seen how the excesses of nineteenth-century medicine finally so dispirited many doctors that they looked outside chemical medicine to techniques such as osteopathy and chiropractic. Within so-called scientific medicine, too, there was a major turning away from poisons. The model was again Paracelsus. For he had never dreamed that the poisons he had introduced into therapeutics would be so recklessly abused. His principle was refinement, and this simple idea was developed in the nineteenth century into a major medical movement.

It fell to a young German doctor from Meissen to make a new interpretation of the theory of 'essences'. Born into a poor family, Samuel Hahnemann made his way through medical school by teaching Greek, Arabic, Hebrew and other languages in which he was unusually gifted. Like Paracelsus, he was soon disillusioned with the medicine of the day, and became a wanderer, 'that I might no longer incur the risk of doing injury'. His only means of support was reviewing and translating medical books, but in so doing he made his fundamental discovery. An English author had attributed the action of quinine to its bitterness and astringency. Hahnemann was certain that these qualities, which were stronger in other drugs that had no effect on malaria, could not be the answer, and he decided to conduct an experiment. He took Peruvian bark himself, and contracted some of the symptoms of malaria. From this and other 'provings', as he called them, he enunciated the first principle of his new system: what cures a sick person produces the same disease symptoms in a healthy person. He called it 'homeopathy', after the Greek for 'same disease', and he lumped all other medicines under the name 'allopathic', signifying treatment by something 'other' from the disease.

Hahnemann then began a search of the literature for examples of poisoning, and experimented for seven years with provings of the effects of various substances on healthy individuals. Thus armed with his own catalogue of treatments to match thousands of combinations of symptoms and patient characteristics, he went back to practising medicine. Cures were claimed, but to avoid the aggravation of symptoms that often occurred at the outset he was obliged to reduce his dosages to one-tenth, then to one-hundredth. It was the Paracelsan idea, but it wasn't working; it was the old problem of finding a dose strong enough to cure without strong side effects.

What has been described so far is what most people remember about homeopathy: treating with ever-diminishing doses of medicines that are 'like' the disease. What is usually overlooked is Hahnemann's solution to the side effects dilemma. The reason for this attitude may be that this solution has overtones of mysticism, but here it is: Hahnemann discovered that his weak dilutions could be 'potentised' by being vigorously shaken. These 'succussions', as he called them, showed that the dynamic action of medicine 'is almost purely spiritual'. For it was contrary to scientific expectations: he could reduce the active ingredient to a single molecule (as we would now call it) – or even nothing – and it would be more effective, after shaking, than a toxic poison.

Hahnemann's writings now begin to take on a Paracelsan sound. The body obviously must have more than an inert, mechanical principle; it must have a 'vital force' and every illness must be a 'cry

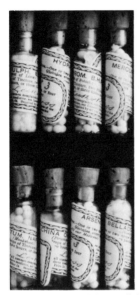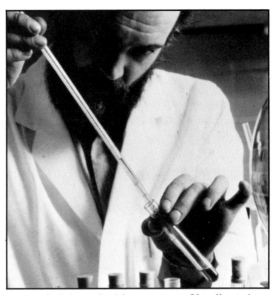

Left. Homeopathic medicines are administered with great care. Usually patients must avoid taking strong drugs and must leave at least half an hour after eating before dropping a pill into their mouth to dissolve under the tongue

Right. Preparing the infinitesimal dilutions of homeopathic medicine. Each substance goes through many stages of dilution and 'succussion', a sharp, shaking technique, before being incorporated into pills

for remedy' corresponding to it. There is a resonance between the body and the remedy. 'The dynamic action of medicines is almost purely spiritual.' Whatever the theory, homeopathy gathered adherents because it worked, especially when compared to the often bungling medical practice of the day.

'Why not put a drop of medicine in Lake Geneva?' the critics hooted. 'Only if I could shake the lake vigorously sixty times,' Hahnemann retorted. In 1812, a typhus epidemic carried back from Russia by Napoleon's army was seemingly kept under control by homeopathy, while bleeding and the use of mercury fared far worse. The same was true of the Asiatic cholera epidemic that swept Europe in 1832. Hahnemann established a school in Paris, his students spread throughout the world, and this treatment rooted in paradox became the choice of the well-to-do, the literary and artistic élite, and finally royalty. In the United States at the turn of the century one in every six physicians was a homeopath.

As conventional medicine cleaned up its act, so to speak, the appeal of homeopathy faded. In the early twentieth century scientific medicine finally began to come into its own. The rational framework of vaccines and powerful, pinpointed antibiotics stood in stark contrast to the 'less is more' incantations of homeopathy. Nevertheless results speak for themselves, and, like the tortoise gaining on the hare, homeopathy is again making an impact as the shortcomings of drugs, their side effects and their disease-specific limitations grow more obvious. The National Health Service includes doctors who practise homeopathy, and there are several homeopathic NHS hospitals. Many members of the royal family use homeopathy. Since 1965 the French government pharmacopoeia has included the preparation methods for homeopathic medicines.

Clinical trials by today's standards have never before been attempted, but are now under way in several countries. An interesting but inconclusive test was made in Chicago in 1884 at the Cook County Hospital – virtually the only comparison available in the literature. Every fifth patient entering the hospital was turned over to a homeopath for treatment. Out of some 6000 patients those receiving homeopathic therapy recovered at a slightly better rate than the rest. For these large numbers, this result is impressive as a general vindication of homeopathy, but perhaps the absence of treatment would have done as well. Additionally, the criterion for 'recovery' would have to be refined.

The best gauge today of the qualities of homeopathy is to compare the experience of going to a homeopath with the conventional doctor's visit. Imagine sitting down for an hour facing this type of questioning. Do you have a tendency to scold? Do you fear you may go insane? Are your feet often damp and cold? Are you unusually neat and clean, or sloppy? How are you affected by music? Are your aches mostly on one side or on the other? Do you have any particularly strong cravings or aversions regarding specific foods? What position do you usually sleep in? Where are your arms when you sleep? Do you stick your feet out from under the covers?

Minute details fill the pages until a portrait of your entire person emerges. Then the search begins to match your picture and your malady with the medication that has matched a similar picture before, as recorded in tome after tome of *materia medica*. Hahnemann himself gives this simple example. A forty-two-year-old business clerk has been ill for five days – first vomiting at night, then sour vomiting for two nights, then a sensation of food that would not digest. He is pale, weak, eager to please, mild-mannered. On questioning, Hahnemann finds that the man also feels his head is vacant and noises of any kind bother him. Hundreds of substances produce

80

vomiting. Like a police inspector, Hahnemann narrows them down: only some substances cause vomiting at night, and fewer yet sour vomiting. Of these, he discovers in his remedy files, only two or three give the feeling of food lying on the stomach. Further winnowing: that vacant, hollow sense in the head eliminates another substance. Intolerance of noise reduces the possibilities to one. The drug is pulsatilla! It seems especially indicated because it matches with non-assertiveness. Hahnemann prescribes half of a quadrillionth of a drop. The next day the patient is fine. Of course it's anecdotal – one of only two case histories reported by Hahnemann, but it's the stuff of medical investigation since Hippocrates, and before. Some would argue that it mimics science without actually being science. For example, a patient with intercostal *Herpes zoster* might have an eruption whose pains are similar to those caused by a bee sting; the homeopathic remedy is an infinitesimal dilution of bee venom. Another person has the same herpes infection, but his pains are worse at night: a variable has been added that describes a person suffering from a toxic clash with arsenious anhydride. A tiny drop of that poison is the prescription. In short the homeopath treats the symptom configuration rather than the disease, and often it is a seemingly insignificant symptom that provides the key to the choice of treatment.

Our sense of time has a funny way of biasing our opinions of various medical approaches. Newer is better, we assume. But the story of Paracelsus, a man out of his time, and the varying fortunes of homeopathy should forever dispel the idea of a linear progression in medicine. Even today's 'magic bullets', those proprietary drugs with names dreamed up by advertising agencies, are often duds.

When annual reports are issued on the progress of health care in Western countries, two statistics are generally cited: infant mortality and life expectancy. In Great Britain and the United States there have been major improvements in ante-natal care in the last few decades, especially among minorities. Accordingly, infant mortality rates have steadily gone down. Life expectancy, on the other hand, appears to be reaching the top of an upward curve, at about seventy years for men and slightly more for women. It is partly the vaccines against the great epidemic-causing diseases but mostly the general upgrading in living conditions that are primarily responsible for this at-birth improvement; and for males in middle age, life expectancy has not improved nearly as much. In both these statements we see indications that drugs do not significantly prolong our lives. Many people have argued that the biblical three score and ten is a rough biological clock that will not be nudged much higher, even by Herculean efforts. The question, therefore, is this: Can drugs help us live *better*?

A nineteenth-century American religious group, the Shakers, had a life expectancy of seventy-one years – about twice that of the surrounding population at the time. By all accounts they lived productive, if protected, lives, and incidentally made part of their living by selling herbs. They had all the lifestyle advantages – diet, exercise, clean environment – of the best communities today. The question arises again: Did they need drugs?

Are drugs helpful to us in those two great traumas that together account for some two out of three deaths in the developed countries – cancer and heart disease? In the latter, drugs have certainly prolonged lives, perhaps compensating for those dietary and lifestyle abuses that are now thought to be the major culprit in early heart attacks. In the case of cancer, the matter is not so clear-cut. With the help of new surgical techniques and improved radiation therapy, certain rare forms of the disease now have high remission rates. The American Cancer Society estimates that roughly half of all cancer victims can be cured. But a disturbing study by Hardin Jones of the University of California has yet to be challenged: his conclusion was that in terms of survival times there is no significant difference between properly matched samples of treated and untreated cancer patients.

The term 'chemotherapy' is used nowadays only in connection with cancer treatment, although it is simply a long word meaning drugs. In this sort of therapy the dilemma that faced Hahnemann has reached frightening proportions. The poisons capable of killing cancer cells of necessity damage surrounding tissue and usually have systemic side effects as well. The controversial laetrile, made from apricot stones, has as its active ingredient cyanide. The hope of new research in this field is that monoclonal antibodies can be targeted solely to the 'errant cells' in the patient.

The man who coined those telling phrases, 'magic bullets' and 'chemotherapy' in German, was Paul Ehrlich. He was born in 1854, almost four centuries after Paracelsus, but he had an uncanny resemblance to his forebear. He was a beer drinker and cigar smoker with a coarse bedside manner. He also had a significant hobby which, like Paracelsus' love of metals, was one of the two 'lines of thought' that would lead to fruitful developments. Ehrlich was fascinated with dyes. He noticed in medical school that methylene blue stained only the nerve endings when injected into the veins of rabbits. He imagined a chemical that could similarly course through the body to just the right place – a magic bullet. It would be specific to a disease, as Paracelsus had contemplated, but would not harm surrounding tissue. It is important to remember dates here. Jenner had successfully vaccinated a young boy against smallpox in 1796 – an experiment with a human subject, incidentally, that would be considered unethical today. Eighty years later, Pasteur laid the theoretical foundation of this practical achievement with the unveiling of the world of germs. Pasteur was to go on to establish the science of immunology, and in 1882 the pioneer German physician Robert Koch was to discover the tubercle bacillus. But in 1875, when Ehrlich began his experiments, there was nothing to suggest a direct cure for infectious diseases.

The young Ehrlich turned to full-time research, obsessed with the idea of giving medical practice a real arsenal of therapies. With the newly discovered aniline dyes he made important contributions to the theory of the immune system; but at the turn of the century he turned his attention to microbial infection, especially syphilis. He moved his laboratory from Berlin to Frankfurt, to be nearer his Jewish patrons and the dye factories, and announced, 'If I have a dye to cure a mouse, I shall find one to save a million men.'

Ehrlich brought two specialists from Japan, Hata and Shiga, to help prepare the experimental animals, mice infected with a microorganism similar to syphilis. Then began the painstaking trials; day after day, slight modifications of an arsenic compound derived from dyes were tried. Occasionally, mice would appear to be cured, but side effects would appear. Further modifications were made to avoid the jaundice, or the blindness, or even more fearsome outcomes. The years passed, but Ehrlich and his team persisted. We take his results for granted today, but Ehrlich's contemporaries thought he was insane to hope for a poison that would single out a disease without causing widespread harm to the body. The 606th attempt also seemed fruitless, but Ehlich discovered a routine error. 'My dear colleagues,' he said, 'for seven years of misfortune I have one moment of good luck.' The drug was dihydroxyarsenobenzene dihydrochloride, happily renamed salvarsan but more appropriately referred to as simply 606. The first human trials, at a hospital in Berlin in 1910, cleared up syphilitic lesions on vocal chords in a matter of days. Patients who had lost their voices could speak again.

Later it was found that in advanced cases 606 produced damaging side effects. Ironically, in these cases doctors had to resort to mercury-chloride, a drug prescribed some 400 years earlier by Paracelsus!

Ehrlich had indeed opened up the modern age of chemotherapy, a word he applied for the first time to disease-specific drugs. A quarter of a century would pass before another major breakthrough would occur. Typically, research now focused on a germ theory for every malady – including pellagra, which had already been clearly correlated with diet. (Insulin had been isolated in the meantime, in Banting's physiology laboratories in Toronto in 1921, but this hormone is not, of course, anti-bacterial.) It was at a dye factory, IG Farbenindustrie, that sulfa drugs were discovered in 1935; but even these were only bacteriostatic: they merely controlled the germs until the immune system could overcome them. Shortly afterwards came the development of the powerful bactericide penicillin. Ten years earlier Alexander Fleming had suggested that the bread mould *Penicillium notatum* might be a good bactericide after noticing that it had eaten away at a culture he was about to discard.

Of the 200 most common drugs used today, only nineteen were developed before 1940. The Second World War provided not only incentives – for discovering quinine substitutes, for example, for the large numbers of troops going to areas in which malaria was still endemic – but also funding for research. It was no longer a matter of a single persistent researcher in a white coat. Merck, a large pharmaceutical firm, examined 100,000 soil samples between 1939 and 1943 and came up with streptomycin, the first successful drug response to tuberculosis. In 1945 came aureomycin (Lederle); in 1947 chloramphenicol (Parke Davis), for use against whooping cough, typhoid and typhus. It also took ten years for cortisone, isolated by Kendall at the Mayo Clinic in 1935 and still the strongest drug against rheumatoid arthritis, to reach the market. The 1960s saw the rise of psychoactive drugs for an increasingly jumpy society: Valium, Librium, Equanil, and the stronger thorazines and chlorpromazine. Who can keep track of them all? A new anti-hypertensive drug seems to come along every few months, and government agencies are speeding up approval times. Biochemically engineered drugs, mimicking various substances produced naturally in the body, have now been passed for human use.

Is the drug approach that our society has apparently embraced the ultimate answer or just another crest of a wave? The drug industry as well as public interest groups and the government all recognise that problems will be encountered and that, however well tested, drugs can go horrifyingly wrong. In the late 1950s thalidomide, a drug given to pregnant women, resulted in deformed babies. Perhaps even more insidious was the case of Practolol (Efaldin), introduced by ICI in 1970 for angina patients. It was hailed as the perfect drug – exhaustively tested on animals and more than 2000 persons over three years. But by 1974 reports began coming in of side effects, notably eye damage ranging from dried-up tear ducts to blindness. An eminent pharmacologist at Johns Hopkins University in Baltimore warns, 'Many of the drugs now on the market have a potential for causing difficulty that is incompletely appreciated.' Even 'safe' penicillin causes twenty deaths a year in Britain.

And there are other considerations. Physicians rightly become nervous at the prospect of facing daily changes in the drug supply line. For example, the November 1980 MIMS, the *British Monthly Index of Medical Specialities*, mentioned sixty new products, eighty deleted ones, forty-three new forms, forty-one discarded forms, and twenty-one changes in warnings or special precautions. Doctors also are aware of iatrogenic illness – caused by doctors. One study in the United States blamed a prestigious research hospital for one disease in every five patients, half caused by drugs. (Very few of these diseases were serious, but most needed treatment.)

This is the face of medicine we have chosen to live with. Having seen it at first hand, I know that medical doctors in China and India can be even more drug-happy than we are. We have also chosen to live with the noise and smell of road traffic and with agricultural pesticides. Automobile accidents are far more injurious to health than all drug side effects. No system of medicine is perfect; all we can expect is an honest exploration of its potentials and limitations.

Ultimately, the stories of Paracelsus, Hahnemann and Ehrlich are the sagas of human beings stretching beyond the visible and expected. While unfinished, their struggle for the enchanted remedy is about the mystery of hope that feeds all healing. Their quest reminds us of Paracelsus' last words that conclude Robert Browning's poem:

> . . . If I stoop
> Into a dark tremendous sea of cloud,
> It is but for a time; I press God's lamp
> Close to my breast; its splendour, soon or late,
> Will pierce the gloom: I shall emerge one day.
> You understand me? I have said enough?

6·THE·MIND·WANTS·BACK·IN

We all know it is possible to blush at the mention of a single word or name. We will even admit to attempting to ease a pain in a sore muscle by closing our eyes and contemplating something pleasant. But we may boggle a little at the idea of influencing the roll of the dice with our minds, and it's definitely unacceptable to pretend to control events 10 miles away. As Dr L. J. Rather of Stanford University points out, the mind-over-matter problem seems to recede the closer we get to home, and in fact endless arguments on this subject are often settled by reducing the mind–body polarity to a mind–brain one, neatly tucking it away in the skull.

If action at a distance offends our sense of reality, then perhaps the mind we speak of is not something lodged in or near the brain, but is an extension of what we call our body. In short, I am a person, not a composite of a physical thing and a mental thing.

Throughout recorded history there have been dualists and monists, yet the concept of an integrated mind–body was generally taken for granted. Aristotle, like the ancient Chinese and Hindus, neatly defused it by spreading the thinking processes around the body, with the heart foremost and the brain very secondary. In the eighteenth century, fuelled by the progress of the natural sciences, the issue began to heat up. La Mettrie's *Man a Machine* staked out the territory clearly: the mind *is* the brain, he declared, and the brain is just another gear in the clock. By the early nineteenth century this soulless view of man was accepted as the scientific model. It was therefore silly to speak of the emotions causing or curing illness, let alone of someone healing himself by sheer force of imagination or will. The ruling powers of the day convened boards of enquiry, much like religious inquisitions, to expose publicly those who would suggest any power of spirit in medicine. But let us look first at how drastically the situation has turned today in the modern medical world, supposedly based so firmly on hard data.

At Harvard University's Beth Israel Hospital, Dr Margaret Caudill conducts a six-month programme for hypertensives – patients with varying problems of high blood pressure – with an agenda that she herself could not have accepted six years ago. From a background in infectious diseases, she tells me, she always expected to work with quantifiable data: blood and urine tests, well-documented protocols. Now she is doing things that she used to call immaterial, the ministrations of yogis.

Her typical patient is a successful middle-aged man such as the one I met – a forty-five-year-old restaurant owner with a ruddy face and impatient expression. His belt was as overworked as he was, for despite his hard efforts and long hours his job was essentially sedentary. He would buy produce before dawn, do the accounts after everyone else had gone home, and toss and turn all night, worrying about – his health.

His family doctor had told him that he had all the signs of impending heart disease: blood pressure of more than 160 over 100, cholesterol reading of 280, high triglycerides and uric acid. He was also concerned about other risk factors: his father had had a heart attack in middle age. The immediate prescription from his doctor was one to alleviate his hypertension. But he was 'lousy and tired', he said, from the beta-blockers and diuretics, and he thought they were sapping his sex life.

So he was here. . . meditating! He was being trained to learn to regulate his blood pressure with his mind, to put it baldly. He would also learn how to relax and to eat things that were better for him. These days Dr Caudill has a different kind of relationship with her patient: her role has become the more passive of the two.

On the first day each participant was attached to a monitoring device indicating blood pressure. Without warning Dr Caudill asked the restaurant owner to tell the group something personal and revealing about himself. He was astonished to see his little black line jump. Already he was beginning to believe there might be something in the idea of a mind–body connection.

Nor did he ever give breathing a second thought. What was there to know about it? Dr Caudill explained that we breathe from our diaphragms when we are babies, and then forget about it in our haste. We start taking short breaths from the upper chest, which adds to tension, which in turn speeds our breathing again. Runners practise 'deep breathing' in full stride; before natural childbirth, women work for months to perfect it.

Dr Caudill said she could always tell when someone was skipping their meditation practice at home: their blood pressure didn't go down. She is careful to confirm her observations, and also her occasional lack of success. She knows that for the great majority who try the programme, which includes a special diet and other techniques devised by the man who baptised and popularised the relaxation response, Dr Herbert Benson, it works.

Why this restaurant owner can gradually wean himself off the drug bottle is the question I hope to answer in this chapter. The monumental work of Dr Hans Selye in Montreal, going as far back as the mid-1930s, is the basis for current scientific attempts to construct an explanatory model. This work on stress has recently converged with the great advances in the theory of the immune system, and a new science has emerged, called psychoneuroimmunology. Evidence is accumulating so fast that a recent reference work in the field, *Mind and Immunity*, lists 1450 abstracts. With the enormous, detailed knowledge we now have of the nervous system, the hormonal system and interactions within the cortex, we are searching for mechanisms that seem much more complex than any dualism, or simple dichotomy between the mind and the body. The case was put most directly by Carl Jung:

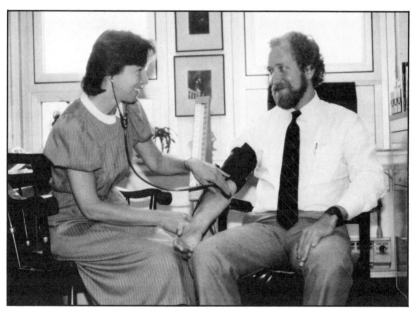

Dr Margaret Caudill taking a patient's blood pressure to monitor his progress under a regime of diet, stress reduction, meditation and exercise

A suitable explanation or a comforting word to the patient may have something like a healing effect which may even influence the glandular secretions. The doctor's words, to be sure, are 'only' vibrations in the air, yet they constitute a particular set of vibrations corresponding to a particular psychic state in the doctor. The words are effective only in so far as they convey a meaning, or have significance. It is their meaning that is effective. But 'meaning' is something mental or spiritual. Call it a fiction if you like. None the less it enables us to influence the course of a disease in a far more effective way than with chemical preparations.

What a different conception of disease permeated the medical profession in the late eighteenth century. Science was the new plaything, and its 'invisible forces', such as Newton's celebrated gravity and Benjamin Franklin's electricity-from-on-high, seized the imagination of the public. What would the next revelation bring? Galvani's frogs' legs moved by electrical current, von Humboldt's idea of the moon exerting a magnetic attraction on earthlings, or further explanations from Newton about this 'most subtle spirit which pervades and lies hid in all gross bodies'? People were going up in hot-air balloons over Metz, the thirteen states had formed a new country in America, and the French Revolution was just around the corner. If man could fly and unlock the secrets of matter, Reason would soon be king. Where was Mind?

Newton's 'subtle spirit' of gravitation sounds like 'mind' or 'soul' to us, but it was all science. A Viennese physician, Franz Anton Mesmer, found himself trapped by this paradox. In 1775, as an expert in the natural sciences, he was summoned before a commission in Bavaria to show that certain infamous 'miracle cures' of his time could be duplicated by science. The cures were all the rage of Europe: a pious German priest was 'exorcising evil spirits' in the name of Jesus and thereby clearing headaches, healing wounds and making crippled limbs usable again. Father Gassner's village church in Switzerland was the Lourdes of its day, but despite the certification of cures by dignitaries of church and state, by noblemen and men of science, jealous protests flooded Rome and the priest was summoned along with Mesmer. The subsequent demonstration unwittingly inaugurated the new field of what we may call 'mind healing', mesmerism or, narrowly, hypnotism.

Mesmer did his job well. He paraded patients in front of the commission, elicited symptoms of illness in them with the touch of a finger, then 'cured' them. He ended his demonstration by praising the priest for his pious faith, but assuring him that his cures were totally explainable by science. They were due, he said, to 'animal

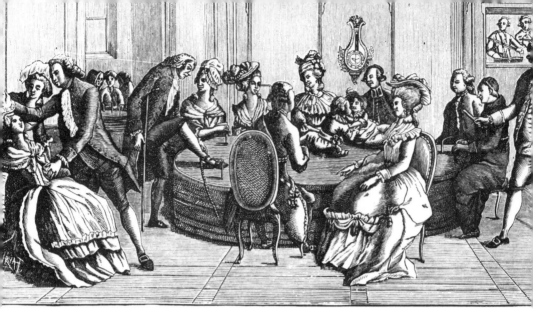

MESMER'S TUB;
Or, a Faithful Representation of the Operations of Animal Magnetism.

magnetism'. The priest was asked to retire to an obscure hamlet.

For his part, Mesmer was launched on a new 'scientific' career. He moved to Paris and expounded his theory of the subtle invisible fluid that fills the universe, connecting people with each other and with the stars. Disease was said to be the result of inadequate supplies of the magnetic fluid. His job, and that of a true doctor, was to restore the equilibrium of fluid among people and, inevitably, all things. His salon flourished, attended by the aristocracy and the Queen herself. Cures were in due course recorded. Sceptical though we may be of Mesmer's rationale, we have to stand in awe of his obvious powers, especially showmanship.

His technology consisted of several large tubs, modelled on the newly invented Leyden jars (predecessors of modern storage batteries), each containing bathwater tinged with iron filings; and movable tubular arms within easy reach of patients for topical application of the ferrous bath, which was neatly stored in bottles emanating from the centre of each tub, like spokes. Patients sat around the tubs, often linked in a full circle, index finger to thumb, in order to 'communicate' the fluid in an 'electric chain'. Portable tubs were available to take home, but Mesmer's house provided the ambiance of a seance. The motion of the fluid was coaxed by the tinkling of a glass harmonica, a pianoforte and 'magnetised' flutes. Overhead mirrors caught the ethereal eddies of liquid through the dim light. Patients waited in expectant silence for a 'healing crisis' to strike one of them – a shiver, perhaps, or a fully fledged spasm of screaming, contortions and collapse. Attendants whisked the fallen to an adjoining mattress-lined room for recovery. For stubborn cases, Mesmer himself would glide into the room in a lilac robe and deftly dispense the fluid on to the uninitiated with a wand or his tapered fingers.

Mesmer's popularity and exorbitant fees did not please the reigning medical orthodoxy. At last Louis XVI was prevailed upon to investigate the man who had unseated Father Gassner. The tribunal consisted of the chemist Lavoisier, who discovered the nature of oxygen, Guillotin (the inventive physician whom the king might well have thought twice about), the leading astronomer Bailly and the American inventor and ambassador to France, Benjamin Franklin. The commission concluded that animal magnetism was a pure fiction, undetectable by scientific means. Evidence of cures was dismissed as the result of 'imagination', and, of course, this was too insubstantial for the newly emerging science to deal with. The panel had in effect decided that mind was a very small thing, and they now pleaded that it be reduced to nothing.

So scientific medicine moved on, continuing to bleed, puke and poison the sick. Disgraced, Mesmer left the field of battle, but his legacy can be traced from one practitioner to the next down to our present-day healers such as Dr Benson, the director of the Beth Israel Behavioural Medicine Department. One of Mesmer's followers, the Marquis de Puységur, noticed that some of his patients entered a strange, trance-like state in which they seemed more aware than when awake. He called it 'magnetic sleep' – magnetism was as fashionable a topic then as are computers today. In 1843 the English surgeon James Braid dubbed it 'hypnosis', after the Greek god of sleep. There was considerable speculation about its mechanism, even though many practitioners became adept at inducing it. A pioneer in the field, Bernheim, was a teacher of Freud; ominously, he theorised that hypnosis was merely an example of a much more common phenomenon, suggestion.

It is to the credit of French medicine that hypnosis was accepted there before the end of the nineteenth century. It was only in the 1950s that it moved out of the theatre and into general use in Britain and the United States. Hypnosis is now known to be a useful, safe tactic in changing stubborn habits such as smoking, over-eating and nail-biting, in treating insomnia, asthma, anxiety, sexual disorders and digestive problems, in promoting a sense of self-esteem and confidence, and in softening the pain of childbirth, menstruation and even surgery. I am aware of cases in which haemophiliacs have been able to control excessive bleeding during an operation by self-hypnotic regulation.

There is no question that hypnotism figured strongly in Sigmund Freud's passage into the world of the unconscious. In one of medicine's most famous clinical encounters, Freud and his senior colleague Joseph Breuer were confronted with a sensitive young woman, Anna O., who had hysterical outbreaks leading to paralysis, speech disorders and hallucinations. Her upper body often became so numb that she could move her head only by pressing her hands to her forehead, and she was subject to uncontrollable coughing. Under hypnosis each symptom began to disappear as she talked about forgotten, painful experiences. Her coughing subsided as she related the story of her father's death: at his bedside she had heard music in the next house and wanted to join the dancing. A speech impediment vanished as she described how she had held herself back when scolded for misbehaving. A now familiar word entered the language for the first time: the unconscious. Freud guessed that the conscious will could be dampened by any free-flowing, untrammelled outpouring of the mind. And so we have free association and today's familiar picture of the patient on the couch talking apparently into the air. Mind had re-entered the world of medicine.

In the continuing history of thought, it seems inevitable that no construct can go unchallenged for long. There is a continual interplay of opposing views, even as new insights, such as Freud's, unfold. The elusive images of the Id, the Ego and the Superego, ideas concerning guilt, sexuality and repressions, did not appeal to many theoreticians working along different pathways at the same time. The behaviourists, following the lead of experimenters like Pavlov (the bell rings, and the dog salivates), wanted to find a more mechanical connection between mental stimuli and physical reactions. In the 1960s it seemed important to test the mind-boggling stories of Eastern mind–body interactions under controlled laboratory conditions. The familiar bed of nails became more than a subject for cartoons; there were now stories of yogis being sealed for days in 'airtight' coffins, or being able to stop their heartbeat for long periods of time, and more. Westerners are turning walking on hot coals into a fashionable experience; science wants repeatability and measurability, not religious experiences that come only under special circumstances. Psychotherapy, that process whose name was coined by Bernheim, worked in varying degrees, sometimes not at all.

But people began to take notice of the power of the mind when yogis agreed to be tested by modern laboratory equipment and showed that all sorts of physiological functions could be turned on and off at will. Meditation was the key, and concentration seemed to be the underlying mechanism. But as major universities began correlating the often esoteric practices of meditation with long-neglected Western studies of stress, it became clear that they were on to something. Machines recorded changes in meditating people which were very different from those just sitting quietly or sleeping. The breath and heart slowed down, oxygen consumption and carbon dioxide elimination decreased, the skin's electrical resistance and the intensity of slow alpha waves increased and there were marked changes in hormone levels in the blood. Psychological changes could be noted. Anxiety, hostility and aggression subsided; energy levels, physical stamina and self-esteem improved.

The reductive power of science has to be carefully watched. Little attempt was made, for instance, to capture the evocative meaning of the meditative act. Is there not a difference between a Zen monk concentrating on 'Who I was before I was born' and a Hindu yogi repeating the universal sound 'om'? Or between a Thai monk 'mindfully' observing thoughts arise and disappear, and a Sufi dervish chanting God's name? Or, for that matter, between a Catholic monk praying for forgiveness and a Jew yearning for the Almighty with all his heart, soul and might? Perhaps their experiences will measure the same on the electrocardiograph. But healing, as we shall see in the next chapter, may have more to do with a person's purpose and destiny than with blood pressure and soreness? Does the scientific net measure the water that passes through it, or only the wet mesh?

Good science goes beyond the ropes, or, as Einstein demonstrated by his endless 'mind experiments', advances on the wings of hypotheses. Two of the most productive hypotheses in this field concern the endocrine system and the autonomic nervous system, and are now well advanced as, respectively, the theory of stress and the theory of biofeedback.

What we commonly call stress is not what Hans Selye had in mind when he set out to construct some unified theory of hormonal activity. We are all familiar with the 'fight or flight' reaction set off by the release of adrenalin. The adrenal gland, so named simply because it sits on top of the kidney (ad-renal), is only one of an interconnected system of hormonal factories: the hypothalamus at the base of the brain, the pituitary beneath it, the thyroid, thymus, pancreas and sex glands. Cannon had described the emergency reaction of the adrenals in 1922; in 1936 Selye hypothesised that there is only one type of stimulus that activates the adrenals, whether it appears to us as heat or cold, infections or injuries. It is what the physician means by the common exposure to anything, and Selye called it stress. His surprising guess was that, whatever the source of stress, the body reacts to it in exactly the same way. There may be an immediate reaction, such as inflammation – this he called the local adaptation syndrome. After repeated excitation of the adrenals, however, there is a general adaptation syndrome, a 'resistance' stage. The 'alarm' stage is normal and healthy; the 'resistance' stage can mean the general breakdown of defences, causing anything from ulcers to cancer.

The non-specific response characteristic of stress, Selye showed, is a reaction not only of the adrenals but of all the glands – the hormone producers. Down the brainstem, through the nervous system and bloodstream flow hormones that increase the heartbeat and blood pressure, raise blood sugar, and shoot glucose to the muscles and brain to rev up the metabolism. Very detailed physiological detective work was not Selye's only strength; what he also offered was something that we might even call spiritual. His landmark study of stress ends with a counsel of nothing short of love as man's answer to a hostile world; we must learn to surrender, to avoid defending ourselves at every turn.

Similarly, the process we now call biofeedback and study with electrodes was first practised and explored in a systematic way by yogis, and had spiritual implications. The control that the yogi exercises over his heartbeat was seen as a form of integration with nature. Before the 1950s, science assumed that the cortex and the subcortex of the brain were not connected – as neat a separation of mind and body as could be imagined. The cortex corresponds with the 'higher' activities of the brain, such as thinking and remembering; the subcortex controls the involuntary, autonomic nervous system – such things as breathing, blinking, pumping blood and muscle contractions. It was then discovered that the cortex was connected to its 'lower' half by a column of cells known as the reticular system. As a result everyone agreed that the cortex indeed needed some of those 'lower' activities merely to focus attention, and probably also to be able to write the letters of a word in the right sequence, to read, and to reason. It was like a two-way street: the cortex was now known to be able to look into the subcortex and make some adjustments.

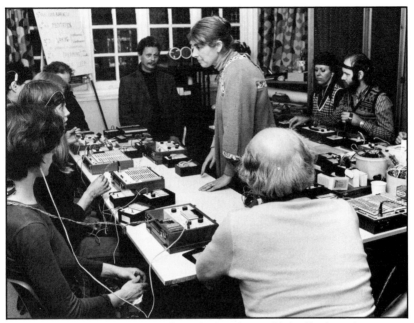

A group of students testing the effect of relaxation on biofeedback equipment

But how? The yogis seemed to do it through sheer willpower. Ingenious researchers soon came up with the clue. The best meditators focused on various parts of the body, watching, listening for minute changes. When something seemed to lower the temperature of one hand, they kept doing it; if it didn't, they stopped. Modern technology amplified this 'signal' with electronic monitors, such as the familiar squiggle of lines on the viewer of an electrocardiogram – punctuated by beeps with every beat. The patient is told to watch and listen intently, and 'feed back' to the body those thoughts or attitudes that correspond to slower beats. It becomes a vicious – rather, a virtuous – cycle; as the pulse goes down the patient is pleasantly surprised and stays with the technique he happens to be following. The pleasant surprise alone contributes to improvement. By the mid-eighties the success of biofeedback has been so well documented that it is taken almost without question. It has proved its value in everything from stopping people grinding their teeth to controlling asthma. At the Menninger Clinic in Kansas, Elmer and Alyce Green have reported that they have been able to control a single nerve cell with biofeedback.

An interesting extension of the biofeedback mechanism is the technique which some have called 'guided imagery'. There is no mechanical feedback of data from the improving body – no buzzers and flashing lights. As in biofeedback, the patient is told to achieve a calm meditative state, then to visualise the disease as something repulsive and the treatment as an avenging angel. So far, this closely resembles the technique of visualisation that has been used for decades by athletes, public speakers and stage performers. The difference lies in the intensity of concentration on events within the person, in the conscious will to influence those inner workings, and in feedback from immediate pleasurable feelings or from later relief of side effects or signs of improved health.

A dramatic instance of guided imagery is the work of Carl and Stephanie Simonton in Dallas, Texas. Carl is a doctor specialising in the treatment of cancer, and most recently an acclaimed researcher. A psychologist, Stephanie has contributed significantly to what is known as the Simonton Method. Where appropriate, they treat their patients with the conventional drugs, radiation or surgery. The still unproven premise on which their method of visualisation is based is that many cancers, if not all, can be traced to a breakdown of the immune system. The interlocking of this system with the endocrine system, the autonomic nervous system, and accordingly the brain – to the point where many researchers now speak of all this as one master system – should allow the mind and the emotions to affect favourably or unfavourably virtually every disease. Unfavourable influences have been conclusively and extensively documented, for example in the case of sudden death or illness after the death of a spouse. So why not mobilise the favourable influences?

Carl Simonton believes that the immune system can, in effect, be monitored with 'mental wires'. Their first trial, in 1971, was with a sixty-one-year-old man with a form of throat cancer considered inoperable. He had already lost 30 lb, could scarcely swallow, and had great difficulty breathing. According to medical statistics he had a less than 5 per cent chance of surviving five years to what is considered the 'remission' age. He agreed to a test of the Simonton theory: it was certainly safe. Three times a day the patient attempted to meditate for fifteen minutes on his illness. He would begin by imagining himself in a tranquil environment, under a tree, by a pond. As soon as he felt quite calm, he was to fantasise about the cancer, letting his grim visions come from the worst horror films. Then he was to turn his attention to the clean, powerful light of the radiation therapy. The cancer monsters were being bombarded by millions of tiny energy bullets. Healthy cells were shielded from attack because they were strong and vigorous. His own army of white blood cells would then rush in to mop up, flushing the dead or dying malignancies out of his body. This fairy tale was to be felt intensely by him, even though it might seem silly to another adult.

The change in the patient's health was stunning. Negative reactions from the radiation began to subside, in turn encouraging more intense play acting, or 'wish fulfilment', as a Freudian might say. After a month he was gaining strength and weight. In two months there were no signs of cancer at all. So impressed was the man by this 'miracle' that he began using the Simonton technique on two additional problems: arthritis and impotence, with which he had been afflicted for twenty years. He overcame both.

A single case can always be considered an aberration, a spontaneous cure – meaning that there is no way of knowing what the real reason was. Perhaps the radiation alone would have worked; perhaps he would have been in that 5 per cent who do recover with conventional treatment. These are the euphemisms that hide the understandable cautious scepticism of the researcher. But this was only the beginning of the story for the Simontons.

Hundreds of cancer patients have now been treated by the Simontons. In their first pilot study, 159 patients, with an average expected survival time of twelve months, lived to an average of more than twenty-four months from diagnosis. At four years after diagnosis, sixty-three were still alive, and more than half of these said their level of activity was as good as or better than before treatment. Because patients were self-selected and the study lacked controls, the results are controversial, but they remain suggestive.

The medical literature is now quickly filling with documentation of guided imagery being used in all sorts of illnesses. One unusual case might be called indirect guided imagery, for the 'fantasisers' were rabbits. The report, which came from Ohio State University in 1980, described what was supposed to be a routine study, using rabbits, of the effects on atherosclerosis of a diet high in fat and cholesterol. When the results were being compiled, something appeared to invalidate the test: in one of the batches of rabbits, the expected hardening of the arteries had not occurred. The experimental animals were supposed to be carefully controlled to pre-empt any unintended health benefits. The researchers went back step by step to find the flaw. At last one of the lab assistants admitted to petting and talking gently to the rabbits in that batch. The experiment was repeated – and was confirmed. This sort of mind–body interaction

97

surprises us more than miracle cures, but it happens all the time.

About 9 million people travel to a small village in the southwest of France each year in search of spiritual regeneration, and secretly, for those who are ill, a miracle. They come with a strong religious faith, a belief in the miracles of the New Testament, and the knowledge that Lourdes is a place of authentic miracles. In 1858 a fourteen-year-old illiterate girl, Bernadette, claimed to have spoken to the Virgin Mary on eighteen occasions. Crowds gathered as she talked apparently into the open air, in rapture, then reported on her conversations – things the Virgin wanted for the saving of the world. The heavenly apparition guided Bernadette to unearth a spring of water where there had not been one before, which has become the site of the most famous healing shrine in the world.

Denounced as a pawn in a well-staged fraud, Bernadette became the centre of a raging controversy. Emile Zola dismissed her as a case of delayed puberty and hysteria. The Catholic church was understandably wary of another situation like that of Father Gassner, another exhibition of misplaced piety. Yet after long deliberation a commission of the Holy Office concluded that 'Mary the Immaculate, Mother of God' did in fact appear to Bernadette, and in 1933, fifty-four years after her death, she was canonised.

To guard against potential fraud and to preserve what was considered hard evidence of cures based on faith and divine intervention, the church went beyond its own canonical commission to appoint an impartial body, the International Medical Commission, in Paris, and a medical bureau at Lourdes. Verifying a cure is difficult. Extensive documentary support is required, not just crutches hanging on a wall. Only so-called 'organic' diseases are considered. The screening is so tight and the standards so exacting that nowadays the number of cures per year averages *one*. The process of verification is as conclusive as any phenomena accepted as true. The church's position apparently is that a 'psychosomatic' cure may be good, but doesn't count because it lies in the grey area which we call 'mental'. In today's scientific parlance, on the contrary, 'psychosomatic' is no longer the leper of medicine: it doesn't mean 'It's all in your mind', but 'It's caused or exacerbated by stress or psychological factors'. Some would claim that all illness has a psychosomatic dimension.

Miraculous cures are characteristic of all religions, and they all involve faith. When Mary Baker Eddy slipped on the ice one winter evening in 1866, her spine was so badly injured that she was pronounced near death. She had been sickly all her life, and had tried every form of fashionable therapy from homeopathy to hypnotism, all to no avail. So this desperate New England woman turned to the Bible, and read the story of Jesus and the paralytic: 'Arise, take up thy bed and walk.' She was healed, and founded the religion that makes healing central to its message, Christian Science. All the things of this world are illusions, including illness, she preached; the only real science is the divine knowledge of perfect health and truth.

But no religion claims that faith is theirs alone. This fundamental human quality pervades medicine, and has been studied as part of the healing process. In one remarkable test forty-six candidates for surgery on detached retinas were interviewed about their attitudes towards their disease, their trust in the surgeon, their optimism about the outcome, their reaction to the chaplain, and their general self-esteem and confidence. According to the answers given, each was placed in a particular position on a 'confidence scale'. Without knowledge of these scores, the surgeon then ranked them by 'speed of recovery'. The two scales were directly correlated.

Another eye-opening study, reported by Jerome Frank of Johns Hopkins University, showed that, as with most religious faith, the physical presence of a healer may be irrelevant. Three patients in a German hospital were considered hopeless cases – one with chronic gall bladder inflammation, one with pancreatitis, and one with cancer of the uterus. The doctor in attendance went to a faith healer since nothing else could be done; without the patients' knowledge, this man attempted twelve times to effect a cure, without success. Then the doctor informed the patients that a faith healer who had performed miraculous cures was going to attempt to heal them. After eight days of building up expectations among the women concerned, the doctor announced that on the next three mornings at a precise time the healer would go to work on their cases, in his own myster-ious way, outside the hospital. The doctor chose that particular time deliberately, knowing that the faith healer did not 'work' during those hours. Again, the results are 'anecdotal – but they were specta-cular. Immediately after the three sessions, all three women began to improve. The gallbladder condition completely cleared and the woman showed no symptoms for a year. The woman with pancreati-tis regained her strength, left the hospital, and had no relapse. The cancer patient survived for three years symptom-free.

What is it that nourishes such faith? These isolated examples aren't intended to prove that there is a mechanism with precise characteristics in faith healing – quite the opposite. In Europe, kings often demonstrated their divine right to rule by healing neck lumps with the 'King's Touch'. Sometimes thousands of people at a time would be treated. Mark Twain's comments are interesting:

> Could the footman have done it?
> No not in his own clothes.
> Disguised as the King, could he have done it?
> I think we may not doubt it.

In many religious experiences, close physical contact occurs. The Hindu saint Ramakrishna's healing touch and the Chinese *qi gong* masters' healing hands are quite tangible. In the well-known cures described in the Bible, Jesus first touches the leper and first rubs a paste on the blind man's eyes. The physician who coached the three women about the faith healer was no doubt a powerful physical symbol to them. The point is that whatever makes an impact on the mind seems to work, and the stronger the impact the better. George Bernard Shaw commented that there are no false legs, only crutches, at Lourdes. Cures only work, it seems, when the body has residual recuperative powers that are activated by the mind.

Recently, science has entered the ancient question of hand-healing hocus pocus, adding another possible perspective. In a very recent scientifically designed experiment Dr Janet Quinn of the University of South Carolina showed that healing hands held 4–6 inches from a patient can produce dramatic reduction in anxiety as compared to non-healing hands. Dr Bernard Grad, a biochemist at Canada's McGill University, conducted investigations on a 'Mr E.' who 'claimed to have observed healing in people and animals on whom he had practised the laying on of hands'. In a series of ingenious controlled experiments wounded mice healed more quickly and barley seeds grew faster. Both researchers are seeking to have other investigators repeat their experiments to ensure validity.

Science has adjusted rapidly to the challenge posed by the new revelations of the power of the mind. All the textbooks prior to 1970 routinely reported that brain cells are not replaced as they die. Then Marion Diamond at the University of California, and others, showed that these cells do indeed rejuvenate. Surprisingly, they grow back when we exercise our brain simply by thinking. Consider what that implies: thought actually makes human cells grow. If the mind is co-extensive with the brain and does not have a reality of its own, this is quite a neat bit of pulling oneself up by one's own bootstraps.

7·THE·RETURN· OF·RITUAL

Both faith and ritual are terms borrowed from religion, but they do not signify the same thing. Faith is one of the ways in which people are healed; ritual, among other things, is what makes faith work.

Why are some people affected by faith healers and others not? Why were some saved by Mesmer's magnetic fluid, others by Hahnemann's potentised potions, and yet others by the balance of water and fire? For that matter, why does it seem that penicillin is so dependable? 'Magic bullets' heal, not people, but a particular disease state of people. They are powerful substances that cause change based on physical, chemical and biological laws independent of human will, imagination or belief. Drugs are dependable, repeatable and work most of the time. They have a magical ability to transform an undesirable state to a desirable one. But science is not the only magic that mankind has developed – only the latest, most successful and mechanical form of it. There are other types of magic that require participation, intention and engagement and a non-scientific sense of the sacred and the special. They can coerce and persuade, perhaps not as reliably as penicillin but nevertheless with their own force. And they have much to do with healing.

Ritual is nothing less than magic, and that magic includes the most powerful medicine known, the placebo; it includes myth; and it includes 'the word', my term for the shared experience of the healer resonating with the healed. Ritual is performance using symbols of what is thought to be powerful in the cosmos. This dramatic enactment changes the actual. It is part of all the healing arts, including scientific medicine. These are strong claims, for they seemingly run counter to scientific medicine's rejection of and separation from the subjective. Part of what I will say is that there is more to scientific medicine than science.

It is difficult to make the major mental shift that this statement entails without a shock. Perhaps in comparing the two true stories below you will experience with me the shock of recognition.

In the early 1950s a new treatment for anginal heart pain was being introduced to surgical wards around the United States. It consisted of a dramatic form of surgery, not performed to remove something or to repair something but to shut off a perfectly good artery so that the body would stop being lazy and start using the smaller arteries to feed the heart. Called 'mammary artery ligation', it showed early promise and the procedure quickly gained in popularity. Patients were performing better on exercise tolerance tests, showed a much more stable heartbeat on the electrocardiograph, and needed less medication. The success rate was reported to be 80 per cent, but then some questions arose and a double-blind clinical test was proposed.

In a double-blind test, neither patient nor examining doctor knows if a real medication has been taken or if surgery has really been performed. It is designed to eliminate the subjective element from a test, to prevent the doctor who wants it to succeed from unwittingly looking at the records more favourably, or to prevent the patient from being misled into thinking he is better, or actually being better because he thinks he should be. This is the placebo effect. In a double-blind crossover test the patients with and without the drug switch places a second time around. Obviously, this is not possible in surgery. It is rare, in fact, for any surgical procedure to be able to be tested double-blind. By today's ethical standards this arterial surgery study would not be allowed. Yet in the 1950s it proceeded, primarily at the University of Kansas Medical Center.

A notice was sent out inviting angina patients to apply for admission to a promising new surgical programme. Availability of places was said to be limited, and only those with seriously weakened functioning were accepted. The 'lucky' ones were told that medical scientists would observe the results of these operations closely.

At the hospital each patient was introduced to a team of total strangers, to whom he or she was literally entrusting his or her life. The patient was most dependent on the famous surgeon-scientist, an acknowledged pioneer in his field, resplendent in his white coat and stethoscope. The others accede to him, but they also have their special uniforms and nametags and hierarchy. The patient obeyed them all, undressing when told, eating and sleeping as commanded. The patient had never done this for anyone else in his life. He did not question anything, for he had been told that this was how he was going to be healed.

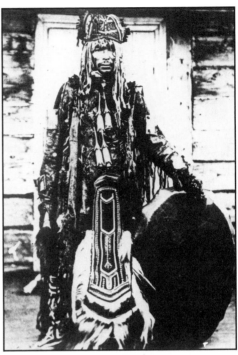

Right. A shaman from Arctic Siberia, a member of the Samoyed tribe. Shamans from this area probably had much in common with the very ancient Chinese ritual and magical medicine that was replaced by philosophic medicines that developed during the fourth century BC in China and elsewhere. The scientific medicine that arose in the West completed this tendency to rationalise medical care

Below. Acolytes surround the Master as he searches for the mysteries of life and death on the operating table

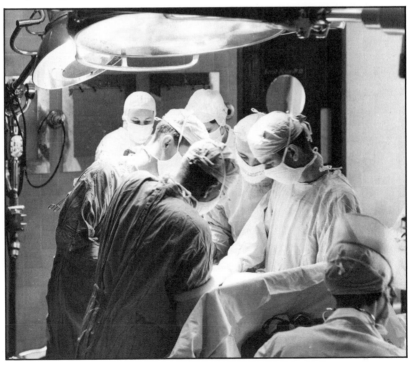

The night before the operation, the procedure was explained again. The patient was told why the surgery was necessary, what dangers it posed. The chances were good but there was no guarantee, and the patient had to sign a paper acknowledging that he knew the risks and was willing to give his 'informed consent', even though that was not yet the law.

In the early morning nurses assembled in his room to shave all the hair of his upper body, to bathe him vigorously with antiseptic soap, to inject him with antibiotics as protection against fever-producing microbes, to ply him with pills to make him groggy and to dry up his fluids, in fact to stun him into passivity. Bottles were strung around him with needles ready to be inserted in him at the proper time. He was then hoisted on to a trolley and wheeled to the operating theatre.

In a special room adjoining the theatre, the team made its last-minute preparations. The surgical team washed and dressed, tied up any long hair, put boots over their shoes and masks over their entire faces, leaving only their eyes exposed. Each one now raised his hands above his head and walked backward into the theatre, spinning around immediately in a dance-like movement to be put into a special gown from attendants. Sterile gloves were pulled over the hands. Each, like a vestal virgin, was now poised for his particular duty.

The patient was now made inert, lifeless, a non-person, with special gases that put him or her into an altered state in which only the involuntary bodily system functioned. The transition to health via a rite that recognises only flesh and blood can only come about if the person is reduced to flesh and blood.

When the body on the operating table was no longer conscious, this was the signal for an index card to be passed to the surgeon. Selected at random, this card told whether the patient should be opened up for artery ligation or merely marked with the scalpel to create a similar scar indistinguishable from that of an operation. The patient had not been told about the cards and the possibility of a sham operation, nor would he be told.

The patient recuperated in the hospital, fully believing that he or she had undergone the life-saving operation. None of the hospital staff except the initiates in the operating theatre knew that some patients had not been operated on. The initiates had been cautioned never to talk about any patient and they were not permitted to see any of them outside the theatre.

One after another many operations were performed and an equal number were faked. The reactions of patients began coming in, from interviews and electrocardiograms. A picture emerged of the difference between the two groups. It didn't make sense: those receiving just the scars were significantly better! The advantage of this group over the group which had undergone surgery was exactly the same by both objective and subjective standards: the fake group had a 40 per cent improvement in its ability to exercise, electrocardiogram and reduction in medication, and a 100 per cent improvement in subjective evaluation of health; the 'real' group had corresponding figures of 30 and 76 per cent.

It sounds like good news: the 'sacred rites' helped both groups substantially. The *American Journal of Cardiology* (April 1960) reported the results with typical enthusiastic comments from members of both groups. But then came the bad news: the mammary artery ligation was considered a failure because it was no better than just giving a patient a scar! No one bothered to look into the reasons for success in *both* cases. The procedure was abandoned. Even if the ritual could improve a patient's ability to walk up the stairs or to reduce his medications and make him feel better, it was not to be done again. It sounds cruel and unscientific, if science means pragmatism. But we are obviously not ready yet for 'shaman surgery'.

In the American southwest lives the most populous native Indian tribe in the USA, the Navahos. Their ceremonies are famous for their colour, intricacy and fervour. Until recently between a quarter and a third of their productivity was devoted to religious chants, and most of that in times of sickness. A Navaho family was willing to pay for the services of the chanters with a substantial amount of its annual income, sometimes several years' income.

How would this tradition deal with a person having the same symptoms as an angina-sufferer? Consider the case of an older Navaho man who feels chest pains whenever he exerts himself and often has shortness of breath. Like the average American, he might rely on self-help measures for aches and pains, stomach upsets and colds, or he would call on his neighbour who had experienced something similar. The Navahos' equivalent of our over-the-counter drugs would be common herbs, which he might search for himself or trade for. There is a Navaho tradition of waiting for things to take their course, saying a simple prayer or trying a sweat bath. But for major illnesses and problems that seem to go on and on, like us the Navaho would go to an expert.

Their diagnostician, our medical equivalent, is called a 'hand-trembler'. The hand-trembler goes to the man's home and asks both him and his family about the illness. The trembler reaches into his bag and produces a 'medicine bundle' made of buckskin and containing coloured gems and stones, painted rods, corn pollen and eagle feathers. These tools will enable the trembler to unite himself with invisible spirit realms, where the significant things in life are decided. The trembler now takes a crystal in his palm, holds it above the patient, and with his eyes closed begins to chant and pray. The drone of the diagnostician fills the small room, as he searches his mind for the cause of the illness. It may have been witchcraft from an enemy, vengeance from one of the gods for not receiving due respect, or retribution for impure ritual or sexual activities. The trembler runs down the list of possibilities, aloud. The animal kingdom is significant: perhaps a coyote had urinated on a rock where the man later sat, or ants trampled by a bear had touched him. Only when he thinks of bats does the diagnostician's hand begin to shake. He senses that the old man has chopped down a tree with bats living in it; and bats have a special significance to the Navahos as the messengers of the spirit world and as teachers. The trembler becomes quiet again, opens his eyes, and prescribes one of the thirty chants known to the Navahos, the 'Hail Chant'. He knows of no other for this malady, and he recommends a specialist, a chanter, the 'Navaho surgeon'.

And so, despite the expense, the family arranges for the chant ceremony in two weeks' time. The tent is cleared and in the four corners oak sprigs and corn pollen are placed. Ritual water is sprayed on the walls, and a herbal fumigation completes the cleansing. Relatives and friends will be invited to partake of little cakes made of the finest corn and resembling hailstones.

The ceremony begins as the sun disappears over the horizon, the symbol of time entering the realm of dreams. From now on there is to be no quarrelling, eating of corn dumplings or, for specifics, urinating facing north. The first two days are consumed in the purification ritual of the sweat baths. Four pokers point out of the fire to the four corners of the earth. Dancing over these, the assembled purify themselves of worldly faults accumulated over a lifetime.

Now it is the patient's turn. He is made to vomit and to clean his bowels by taking herbs. The suds from the soapy yucca cactus clean him, and fragrant herbs anoint him. A cacophony of drums, rattles, whistles made of the largest bone of the eagle wing (to make his spirit soar), and 'bull-roarers' made of wooden slates (to cleanse and strengthen him with their screeching) fill the room. The patient is moved to a public confession of his sins and his violations of taboos. The climax of the ceremony is now about to be reached, and the arena is purified and readied.

The third day begins with a new forcefulness in the drums and rattles. Now the songs begin, acted out with gestures and stances. Reeds are lit – filled with fragrant plants, bluebird feathers and native tobacco – as a sign to the gods. And the patient is identified to the gods by the eagle and owl feathers, as well as snake-like painted sticks, placed on him. The gods are also offered refreshments in the form of cornmeal figurines in the shape of porcupines and snakes. If everything is done precisely the gods will perform their healing act.

The chanter is the key. His songs tell the story of Rainboy, a Navaho hero. Sometimes it sounds like a morality play, at other times like *Star Wars*. It starts with the simple Rainboy, an innocent gambler, getting into all sorts of small scrapes. Rescued by the humblest of the Navaho Holy People, the Bat, Rainboy eventually wanders to a strange land ruled by the White Thunder God, master of the rare winter thunder. Out of nowhere, the wife of White Thunder lassoes Rainboy with a preternatural rainbow, and seduces him. Contorted by jealousy, White Thunder takes revenge. He smashes Rainboy into small pieces, scattering them in all directions. But the other gods take pity on the innocent Rainboy and a war ensues between them, the kind Holy People, and the angry White Thunder and his allies. This cosmic clash creates the Navaho map and their customs once and for all. The battlefield is the sacred space of the Navaho; the only real time is this 'main event'. A truce is finally established so that healing rites can be performed.

The bits and pieces of Rainboy are gathered by the Thunder People and placed between sacred buckskin. White Wind is put under the top cover and Rainboy starts to move but he can't get up. Now Little Wind enters the buckskin bed, giving Rainboy the power to hear and move his fingers. Talking God sends moisture under the covers so that the boy now has tears, saliva, perspiration and the use of most of his joints, but he still cannot arise. Another god blesses him with corn pollen to give him fingernails, toenails and hair. Insect and Spider People gather his blood and nerves. Still something is lacking.

The Holy People decide to undertake the four-day Fire Dance. Each Holy Person performs his own song and dance. Gradually Rainboy's parts become whole, and he emerges from the covers. Now he is presented with gifts: he is to be in charge of rain, mist and

107

holiness, of beautiful birds and the harvest. Once an ordinary mortal, now he is invited to join the Holy People.

Rainboy has made the full journey. He has gone to the Land Beyond the Sky, he has been dismembered, and he has been renewed by fire. Because he has known brokenness, his new intactness is different; because he has died he is now resurrected. But before he becomes a Holy Person himself he must teach the story of his journey and his healing ceremony to his brother and sister, who pass it down to the Navaho ancestors. This ritual of the timeless past is now being re-enacted for the old man, and to make it real the boy-hero himself will be brought to the tent.

So it is that on the fifth day the patient is told to wait outside the tent. Inside, long before dawn, the chanter begins to draw on the floor elaborate pictures made of multicoloured sands, representing the story of Rainboy: his encounters with White Thunder, with the other Thunder People, with the forces who have healed him, with Female Corn, Cornbeetle, God, Frog and Bat, all of whom embody the ultimate power and reality of the traditional Navaho. The chanter spends hours constructing this elaborate picture with pulverised stones of red, yellow, blue, pink, black and white. Unless each detail is correct the ceremony may be worthless or harmful.

As the sun rises the patient is called inside and told to sprinkle cornmeal on one picture and to recite prayers. Then he returns to the centre of the tent; the moment of transformation is at hand. The drumbeats and rattling become intense as the entire community squeezes into the tent. At last the chanter places his moistened hand on the sand picture and solemnly touches the old man. The patient is now one of the Holy People. He repeats after the chanter:

> This I walk with, this I walk with.
> Now Rainboy I walk with.
> These are his feet I walk with,
> This is his body I walk with,
> This is his mind I walk with,
> This is his twelve plumes I walk with.

The drumming, the chanting and the incense-burning continue. The progression of feelings goes from restored health via happiness to beauty. The chants continue all through the sixth day, and on the seventh they reach a glorious climax: 'In beauty I walk. . . . In old age wandering a trail of beauty, living again, may I walk. . . . It is finished in beauty. It is finished in beauty.' He is transformed into a god, and those around him with their own ailments are likely to be healed with him. For several days thereafter the old man stays by himself, leaving his hair unwashed and eating unusual foods. It takes time to return to his former human self, whole again.

I have described these two examples of the ritual of healing in considerable detail so as to make the point that what we see through modern eyes as superstitious twaddle may not be so different from our own rites. Granted, the surgeon does not intend the ministrations of his staff and the aura of his operating theatre to be ritualistic. But to the patient the effect of the smells of strange gases and antiseptics are like incense; the sounds of whirring motors are like drums; the monotonous voices over the intercom are like chants; the gowns and masks are like tribal costumes. The Navaho firmly believes that the chanter knows what he's doing, just as the angina patient has complete confidence in the art and science of surgical procedures. The distinction is that the surgeon has a different viewpoint of how he heals. I don't mean to suggest that fake surgery is an effective or ethical way to deal with disease; my point is that there is a strong ritual element in much of modern medicine. Ritualistic healing is not being squarely faced and examined.

John Powles, writing in *Social Science and Medicine*, asks if the coronary care unit so prominent in 'engineered' medicine is not as ritualistic as 'the magicians of old', in terms of its lack of scientific efficacy. He cites other examples, such as the doctor who knows that an upper respiratory infection is viral but prescribes an antibiotic anyway because his patient 'deserves it'. He knows in his heart of hearts that his patients don't understand the difference between a virus and a bacterium, and may feel better just by being 'treated'.

Is there a way of getting a closer understanding of the potential power these rituals all share? Fortunately, a mass of information on this healing force has begun to accumulate in the most unexpected place, the scientific laboratory. It relates to that controversial subject, the placebo effect.

There is a long literature on the power of suggestion. In the 1920s many attempts were made to improve the conditions of people working in factories, and it was found that virtually any change would improve productivity simply because the workers were being attended to. In medicine, the drug explosion of the fifties began to put extreme pressure on researchers to prove efficacy as well as safety. Double-blind drug studies were introduced. In the United

States, the Food and Drug Administration became notorious for its rigid standards, resulting in what the pharmaceutical companies called the 'drug lag' of five years and often more from the introduction of a new product to its approval and marketing. The way to show efficacy seemed to be to disentangle the 'real' properties, the chemically demonstrable effects, of a drug from the subjective state of the one taking it. As mentioned earlier in connection with sham surgery, this means testing two groups of people, both of whom believe they are taking the drug, though they are aware that they are part of a study. This subterfuge is carried out by creating a fake pill, identical in size, colour and taste to the real pill as far as is technically possible. Like the little sugared tablet given to children to please them, this pill is called a placebo, from the Latin 'I will please'.

In effect science was being asked, in the double-blind test, to confront, evaluate and discard that tiny ritual effect of taking a pill. As described earlier, the word 'double' refers here to the fact that the eagerness of the researcher/doctor to see a cure is also taken into account. The placebo effect implies both 'Wishing will make it so' and 'Knowing the expected answer induces one to see it.'

Herbert Benson and Mark Epstein noted in the Journal of the American Medical Association in 1975 that it was abundantly clear that the effect of the placebo was not only surprisingly strong but also consistent. About one-third of those people taking a placebo would be treated by it as well as if they had taken an effective medication. Strangely, the placebo seems to mimic other aspects of a drug: the better the drug the better the placebo is. It must also be emphasised that when the placebo works it works like the drug – that is, it actually makes physical changes in the body. It isn't that the patient simply believes his ulcer is better – it actually heals; or that the arthritic believes he can walk – his inflammation is actually reduced. Virtually any organ or physiological system in the body can be reached by the placebo effect. Inert though placebos may be, they can affect adrenal gland secretion, angina, blood cell counts, blood pressure, rheumatoid arthritis, vasomotor function, gastric secretion, insomnia, pupil dilation and contraction, respiration, fever, pain of various kinds, the cough reflex and even the common cold. There is nothing in the 'green pharmacy' or in the modern armoury of drugs with such power and versatility.

To see the placebo as simply an example of faith or the power of suggestion would be a mistake. It has a dependability and breadth of application that root it deeply in every healing process from surgery to the shaman, from chiropractic to Chinese herbalism. In attempting to discount its effect in healing, science has documented the technology of magic and displayed it like a wonder drug – which it is. The possible can change the actual.

The placebo works on many levels. It can be enhanced by the patient's perception of the healing performer. In an experiment with bleeding gastric ulcer patients, an inert pill was given to two well-matched samples, in the first case by a senior physician who characterised it as a potent drug; in the second case by a nurse who said that the drug might or might not be effective. The first group had an actual, not imagined, recovery rate of 70 per cent, while that of the second group was only 25 per cent.

Packaging can have totally unexpected effects, too. The small white pill, perhaps because it is so common, performs the placebo effect the worst. The best are multicoloured capsules; if large, they should be brown and green; if small, red/orange or pink. The response also depends on the illness: anxious or phobic patients respond better to green placebos, depressives to yellow ones. If the pill is supposed to be a stimulant, you might guess that red and pink would perform better than blue. It has been shown that brand names like Disprin work faster than those which have merely a generic name like aspirin.

The placebo is a chameleon; it can turn itself into anything the healer wishes it to be, even if the effects are diametrically opposite. Asthmatic patients were told that an inhalant would induce asthma – it did; then they were told that there was another substance that would reverse the attack – it did. Both substances were the same, an inert saline solution. In a famous experiment reported by Stuart Wolf in the *Journal of Clinical Investigation* (again, one that would not be countenanced today), pregnant women suffering from nausea were given syrup of ipecac, which normally causes nausea by stopping stomach motility. They responded as expected, and a small balloon swallowed to enable their stomach contractions to be studied showed that motility had been reduced. The next day the women were given the same drug, but told it would stop nausea. It did, and the balloon showed that the contractions had increased.

As this example suggests, the placebo is far from harmless. In one of the early, double-blind studies of birth control pills, fully 30 per cent of those who took the placebo reported decreased sex drive. In this very large study there were also complaints of headache, increased menstrual pain, and nervousness and irritability. Other drug trials, reported in *The Annals of Internal Medicine* by D. M. Green in 1964, whose purpose was to test for drug effectiveness and not for side effects, have turned up such hard-to-imagine problems as constipation, skin eruptions, palpitations and hearing loss. And several studies have even disclosed the unhappy news that there can be severe withdrawal symptoms after discontinuing an inert pill!

If the placebo is more than the power of suggestion, more than faith in science, or more than distrust of medications (as the negative effects might indicate), just what is it? Science has no answer yet. I think science cannot find an answer, because it is not the sort of thing that science deals with. For science, time is endless, space limitless, values relative and truth progressive. People are interchangeable and there is no room for enchantment. For ritual and myth, some parts of space and time are qualitatively different from others. Connecting to 'sacred' time and 'charged' space is the driving force of magic. Science recognises itself by its separation from such subjective and special experiences, and our medicine men try to keep their distance from the placebo like a duck hunter who has just shot a skunk. The placebo and magic are more like a unicorn; they don't exist on the same level as ducks or skunks. The scientist wears a very special kind of sunglasses that filter out unicorns the way they filter out ultra-violet light. And if a unicorn somehow appeared, science would describe it as a horse with a large bump on its head. But the medical scientist will have to take off the glasses to see what Norman Cousins calls 'the medicine man within'.

In discussing the limitations of modern medicine, Powles suggested a direction we must explore if we are to understand the ritual of medicine that includes the placebo effect. He hints at the tendency of medical science to hold tenaciously to 'engineered' medicine, simply adding on *ad hoc* patches when confronted by something like suffering. He writes:

> The problem of disease cannot be reduced to the purely technical one of the prevention and correction of biological malfunctioning. Nor is it sufficient just to add on the dimension of emotion. . . . For in addition . . . there is the threat that disease poses to be the individual's sense of his own integrity and well-being. This existential challenge, in the ultimate, is the threat of oblivion.

Most recently, Eric J. Cassel has focused on the same issue, the larger dimension of suffering, in the *New England Journal of Medicine*. The actual disease or injury may be only a small part of the pain of suffering, he points out; suffering may also include the fear and the reality of devastating medical treatment, of social isolation, of disruption of life. In general, Cassel defines suffering as 'the state of severe distress associated with events that threaten the intactness of the person'. The philosopher Heidegger calls it 'being at issue'.

What the Navaho diagnostician and the sham-surgeon and the placebo in all its forms have to do with one another is the idea of intactness. It is this reality that the Eskimo shaman, in Claude Lévi-Strauss' famous commentary, 'The Sorcerer and His Magic', eventually stumbles upon. The shaman tells, in a published biography, how he decided one day to infiltrate the ranks of his fellow Eskimos and expose their superstitious shaman practices. The more he learned, the more he realised that the shamans were indeed aware of the qualities of performance in their art. Yet they continued practising their magic because they genuinely believed that they were healing, and that their people would benefit from their rituals. Eventually he became a shaman himself, retaining his scepticism in his cortex but leaving it behind in his healing ministry to his people.

The Navaho 'Hail Chant' described above is a full-blown Wagnerian opera compared to the average scene in a hospital. It has the added trimmings of total community involvement, the cathartic component of confession, some herbal elements, and the sensually transforming force of music, dance, rhetoric and poetry. Is the chanter slightly sceptical of his own performance? Perhaps. But the difference between the surgeon and the chanter comes down to what part of the total healing experience each emphasises. The surgeon sees his healing world as 95 per cent physical and 5 per cent ritual. The shaman sees his world as just the opposite.

It is all too easy for anyone raised in Western cuture to miss the fundamental dimension of life as seen by pre-literate people. The seven-day ritual of the 'Hail Chant' contains the essential Navaho truth, just as the tableau of Adam and Eve conversing with God and the snake in the Garden of Eden defines the identity of some of us. The tribe maintains its sense of intactness by surrounding itself with this vision of what existence is all about, immersed in both a close-to-nature and supernatural experience which we find hard to visualise. The essential content of the story of Rainboy is that dying is at the core of life, that brokenness is the core of wholeness.

Thus the 'Hail Chant' is far more than something designed to create the placebo effect, more than a mindless performance. Just as modern surgery is more than empty ritual and is concerned with removing tumours, attaching retinas and replacing joints, the

113

Navaho ritual has its own real content. It connects the Navaho with his cosmos and allows for an experience of transcendence that can heal.

The myth, if we can call it that, on which biomedicine operates is alien to us. It has no cosmology or meaning. Its forces are just as mysterious to the layperson as academic theology is to the average believer. It presents a face of remoteness and impersonal power, with marvellous terms such as X-rays and ECGs and CAT scans and the nuclear power resonator and positron emission tomography scanner – terms and names which would excite the imagination of Mesmer himself. We must believe that those demons are further barriers to annihilation, but they are not concerned with what is important in our lives. But they never let us get beyond being a bundle of statistics wrapped in human form. Our person-hood appears as an irrelevant spectator. They are incapable of evoking in us what the 'Hail Chant' invokes in the Navaho, the experience of what it means to journey through life, and how that life can have intactness, vitality, cohesion and personal purposefulness. And so we have lost our feeling for the sacredness of the world, and our place in it.

Yet we continue to hold, as human beings must, to fragments of what was once our oneness with the world. Deep within each of us are personal myths that sustain and enrich the drama of our lives. We have sacred places, too: our home town, the place where we fell in love. And special moments: the last moment with a parent, the birth of a child. A sacred meaning need not be pious or cosmic: it can be devotion to organic gardening or skill in embroidery. They are what activates our deepest part, enlists our commitment and connects us to the process of being alive. These personal vestiges of the sacred may not be as strong as the unified myth of a tribal people, but they are what makes it possible to live in a real sense. When we face the threat to our existence, they are what we most fear losing. Medicine that ignores this can never be fully healing.

There is one last lesson we can learn from the Navaho myth: healing ceremonies do not exist solely for redressing suffering. Sickness reaches down into the deep-seated paradoxes of the human dilemma and the healing ceremony is a way to the inner realm of the spirit, what the Navaho calls *biigistiin*, or the one who lies within. We might use the word 'soul'. Illness for the Navaho is the rare opportunity to intensify this journey to a deeper experience. It brings him to the source of his being, so that his brokenness can be transformed into intactness, so that our healing can encompass a reconciliation with our humanity beyond any question of just physical repair.

8·THE·OPEN·CLINIC

One of the most delightful paradoxes in our polyglot world is that it is our diversity that makes us a single human race. The old keeps overtaking the new, the unlearned give lessons to scholars, the sick and the weak inspire the healthy. At the edges of each of our lives exists a friction with other ways of living that ignites the energy that is uniquely human.

In the clinic where I work diversity has been consciously and systematically harnessed to drive a new kind of medical treatment programme. The diversity extends to patients as well as to the range of healing arts explored in this book, and I would like to tell you about those patients and how we work with them.

The hospital of which we are a part, Lemuel Shattuck, is the largest chronic disease hospital in the Boston area. It is run by the Commonwealth of Massachusetts, and named, incidentally, after the founder of public health in America. It is an innovative centre; among its current research projects, for example, are major studies of sleep disorders, cancer of the prostate gland and health problems of the homeless. The hospital's mandate is also to provide programmes needed but not available and our clinic is a pioneering effort at what we call 'full service' health care.

It comes as a surprise to people that we are called a Pain and Stress Relief Clinic. Most hospital clinics are named after types of diseases or therapies. Ours, on the other hand, approaches illness from the point of view of the experience of the patient, regardless of the malady. This is not to say that it is better or worse, but that by focusing on the trauma of the person – his or her pain – it is fundamentally different. One cannot compartmentalise the experience of chronic pain. It always has the dimension of physical pain, mental anguish, behavioural disruption, social dislocation and spiritual suffering. In many ways, this is true for all major illness.

When I say it is 'my' clinic, I mean that I am currently its clinical director. It is my task to make the diversity of our staff a unique benefit to our patients – pushing each practitioner to the boundaries of his or her healing discipline. It is the task of our administrative director, Michael Zucker, to maintain order amid the confusion I sometimes create and to make the practical business of schedules and treatment go forward in a sea of intellectual, therapeutic, emotional, and often linguistic competition. And there are many others who helped found this unique place in 1980 and continue to nourish it.

It probably says more about the clinic's work than anything else that we all know we will go elsewhere when we stop learning. That is not our primary purpose, of course, yet we receive applications from all parts of the world from practitioners who want to work with our staff. We have fewer than fifty practitioners and fifteen supervisors, and when a position falls vacant there are dozens of applications for it. We have young housemen gaining their necessary hospital training in such fields as medicine, psychology, acupuncture, nursing, physical therapy or nutrition. We have students and observers from the major medical schools of North America and Europe. Students from Harvard Medical School mingle with apprentices of shiatsu. We engage in various research studies and are a site for an international cross-cultural study on chronic pain for the National Science Foundation. All these affiliations and activities contribute to the mix of our healing arts and a dynamic and searching environment.

Will a psychiatrist working with an acupuncturist be a different pyschiatrist? A better one? A muddled one? Will a nutritionist develop sensitivities he or she did not suspect existed, by seeing how a hands-on therapist analyses a case? Can one of the Eastern 'movement' practitioners find insights in the work of a physical therapist? How will a vocational counsellor and a Harvard-trained doctor provide a coherent plan for a patient faced with the many dimensions of chronic pain?

Each patient as he or she enters the clinic has only a few things in common with the next person: his age, his income and his sense of desperation. We place a high priority on the elderly; the average age of our patients is about fifty. We never refuse treatment for lack of money. Hospitals refer to us their most difficult cases, the 'tertiary' care problems. Though our waiting list is long, most people are willing to give it one last try; they have been on a treadmill of drugs and doctors and despair for too long. For some, sickness and pain have been almost a career. Some come with exaggerated hopes,

116

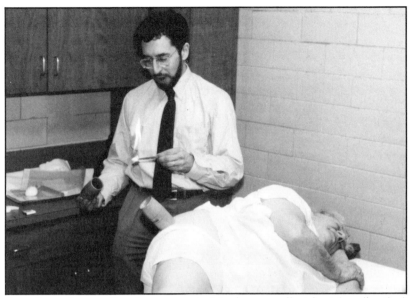

As well as using needles, the acupuncturists also use radiant heat (moxibustion) from burning herbs, and, as shown here, cupping, making a vacuum in a bamboo tube which clings to the skin

others with very few. Some trust us immediately, others wonder about our unconventional therapies. Some are patient, some nervous and belligerent. They are all shattered, and the secret places in their lives are devastated.

I try to see all patients at least briefly in the twelve-hour intake process, but I know there will be time over the first few weeks to get to know them personally. Though I have been surprised many, many times in my clinical work I think I can sense from the start which specialities have the most chance of doing some good in each case. Often it isn't what the patient wants. Confronting pain can hurt. I can predict which therapist will strike a sympathetic chord, what programmes are probably a waste of time, and when a crisis is likely to occur. But human nature is never exactly predictable. I have to fight my own complacency as well as that of some of the staff; I have to end my internal contradictions as well as mediate in disputes and dampen over-enthusiastic proposals.

Since there are more than thirty distinct therapies available at the clinic, steering the patient towards the right ones is a critical procedure. We start with five or six evaluations from the major diagnostic disciplines. Then we confer, and suggest the next direction of treatment – which might involve another five or six therapies. The

117

system is strangely self-correcting. The give and take, the challenge and self-examination sharpen each practitioner in a way that never happens when they are surrounded by carbon-copy colleagues.

Patients begin with the most familiar framework – the standard medical intake. Our examining practitioner knows she probably won't discover anything missed by the X-rays, CAT scans, ECGs or myelograms that other hospitals have taken. The blood count, haemoglobin level, blood pressure and pulse are probably also in the same range as indicated on previous reports. But sensitive questioning is also vital in this high-tech medicine, and our practitioner is highly skilled at it. Armed with electrolyte data, sedimentation rates, pictures of decalcified bones or protruding discs, or measurements of inflamed joints, she interprets the numbers with compassion, explaining that these are ranges that can vary in importance from person to person, that the pain can be dealt with. She is also the necessary link between our clinic and other departments of the hospital, such as neurology or orthopaedics.

Now the patient sees a research psychologist, who has the unenviable task of gathering information about the patient's pain and converting it into hard data. She tries to measure pain, that totally personal sensation, and make it public and unaffected by the social circumstances of the observer. This data will then be used in research or presented to the medical review committee of the hospital to demonstrate the efficacy of our programmes. We want to know the quantity and quality of this person's pain at the beginning, middle and end of the patient's sojourn in our clinic. Also, we need such data one year after completion, to make sure that the benefits of the programme have been maintained. Our patients are a challenge because they are usually the ones who slip through the health-care network – the old, the poor, the helpless and the hopeless. (We tell our new housemen that if they work here for a year they won't be afraid to tackle any patient anywhere; it's not surprising then, that some volunteer to work without pay.) We administer the standard questionnaires that are used in pain clinics elsewhere, to connect with the 'scientific community'. Finally, our psychologist tries to form a picture of the patient's outlook for the benefit of the rest of the staff. Little clues come out in gestures and language. Different types of words, for example, are chosen to describe pain: physical words such as cutting, throbbing and crushing; emotive words such as frightful and terrifying; words full of meaning, such as cruel and torturing.

118

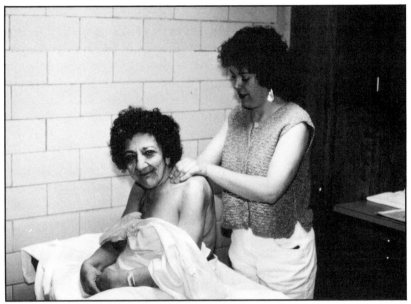

The various types of 'hands-on' therapies available in the Pain and Stress Relief Clinic range through many techniques from physiotherapy to shiatsu

Usually the clinical psychologist or psychiatrist meets the patient next, to go deeper into the personal life of the sufferer. Where in the vicissitudes of life can the pain be located? Is the pain magnified by guilt, anxiety, fear, shame? Is past pain being relived by reacting to bygone events or people as if they were important now? Is depression amplifying bodily sensation to increase pain? Is suicide a possibility?

Current behaviour can also increase pain, and it is the job of the stress counsellor to evaluate this possibility. Pain can be increased by heightened states of arousal or by apparently unconnected events in the patient's home life and medical visits. Behaviour patterns and learned attitudes can include such simple things as seeking excessive attention from others, or holding one's breath, or constantly thinking about pain. By identifying the attitudes and activities that increase the pain, the patient can learn to monitor himself and change that level of sensation, just as in meditation a person can learn to lower his blood pressure. In fact, meditation is one of our main therapies.

The social worker and the vocational counsellor view the patient as the product, at least partially, of his environment. It may be that constant poverty or marriage problems have conditioned the patient to experience pain. A person with a meaningful life generally has a better chance of returning to health than the hopeless individual.

119

Our physical therapist, who is also trained in osteopathic manipulation, sheds light on yet another dimension of the patient – one that is overlooked in a surprising number of cases. The very structure of the body can be pain-inducing in unexpected ways: such things as bodily alignment or posture, muscular weakness, tightness, restrictions in movement. For the physical therapist, the bodily form is the web that holds pain. She, like our movement therapist who uses dance, yoga and *tai chi*, shows the patient ways of being and expression of which they had only a dim idea before.

Our 'touch' therapist lays his hands on the patient immediately; his evaluation comes from his own sensitivity to soft body tissue and inmeasurable qualities like tension. Our masseuse may not add anything new to what the physical therapist has reported, except something about a 'feel', but the patient may see it differently from his or her perspective. In fact, the first step to recovery often begins here. Patients experience for the first time, sometimes in years, what it means to feel good. And later they are taught how to achieve the same effects by themselves.

The most exotic encounter between patient and staff is likely to occur in the office of the oriental medical practitioner. It is a form of culture shock that few patients have faced in their lives. When it is explained that pain results from a disharmony in basic qualities of being, the patient may feel either that he is on to a higher level of truth, or that he is in the presence of a madman. And it is true that the images of Chinese medicine are strange to Western ears. From the descriptions of the opposing forces of *yin* and *yang* – cold and dampness versus heat and wind – one might think one was listening to a weather report of the body. Yet many patients respond to the diagnosis of this system more easily than to a computer printout.

Patients are asked to bring a food diary on their first visit, so that our nutritionist can get off to a good start with this important component of daily life. Here the initial focus is on disruptive eating habits, often a big problem with pain sufferers whose only pleasure can be eating. Later, the nutritionist will have data from which to explore poor nutrition and possibilities of therapeutical alterations in the diet. Also, nourishing and caring for oneself can be an early step out of the 'helplessness' of chronic pain.

The biggest shock to patients is their introduction to other patients in the 'support group'. They have probably never before been surrounded by people in similar situations. They are no longer special or isolated because of their illness, but are brought closer to others who

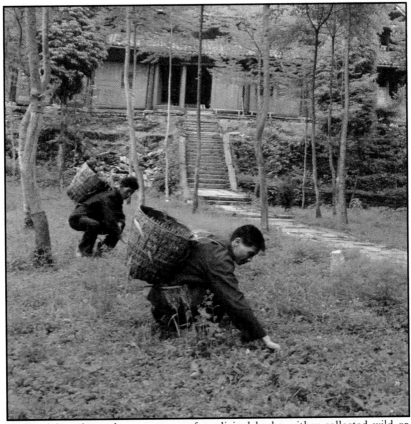

Mt Emei has always been a source of medicinal herbs, either collected wild or farmed. This herb farm is based in a monastery; the trees are grown for their medicinal bark and other herbs grow around them

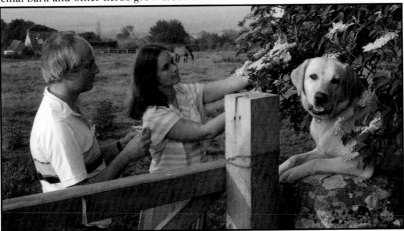

Michael and Ann McIntyre, herbalists of the English tradition

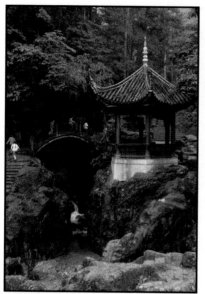

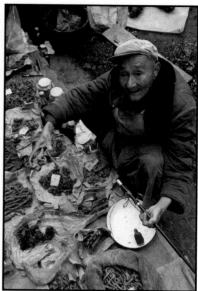

Left. Thousands of Chinese tourists climb Mt Emei, a mountain that was sacred to Buddhism and which still has many monasteries on its slopes where visitors can stay overnight on their way to the 2600-metre summit. The mountain has an extraordinary range of plants, 100 of which are unique to this site

Right. There are stalls along the paths leading up the mountain, where the tourists can buy herbs, antlers, the bones of monkeys and other medicinal substances

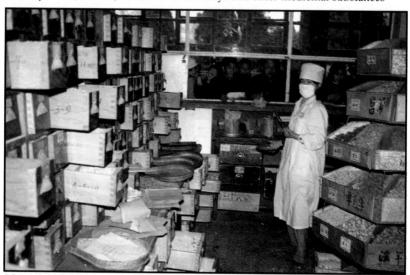

Most of the herbs are gathered from the mountain and are sent to pharmacies all over the country. This one, in Chengdu, contains at least 1000 substances, some considered to be so valuable that they are kept in a safe. This pharmacy is similar to the one in which Ted Kaptchuk worked

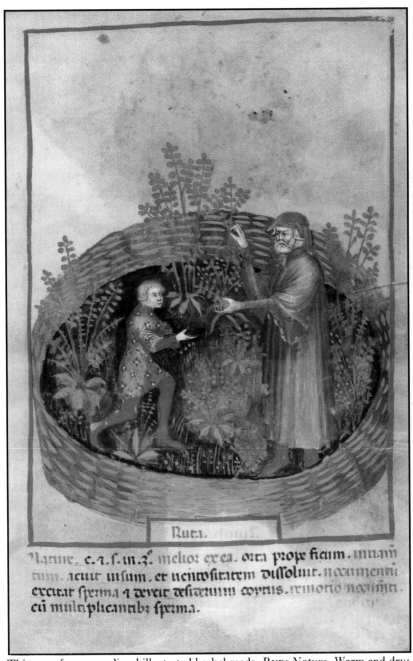

Ruta.

Nature. c. 7. f. in 3°. melior ex ea. orta prope ficum. miuam
cum. acuit uisum. et uentositatem dissoluit. nocumentii
excitat sperma 1 deucit desiderium coytus. remotio nocumii
cu multiplicantibz sperma.

This page from a medieval illustrated herbal reads, Rue: *Nature*, Warm and dry;
Optimum, That which is grown near a fig tree; *Usefulness*, It sharpens the eyesight
and dissipates flatulence; *Dangers*, It augments the sperm and dampens the desire
for coitus; *Neutralisation of the dangers*, With foods that multiply the sperm

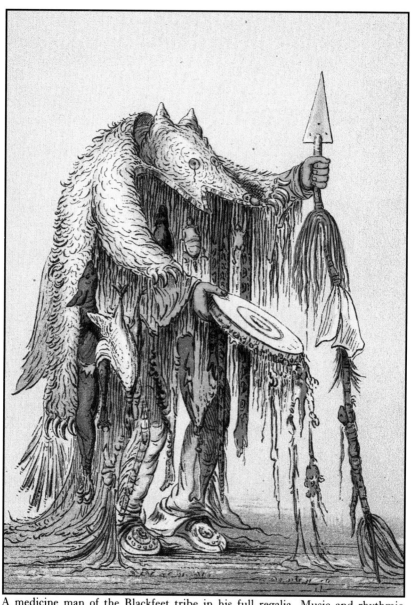

A medicine man of the Blackfeet tribe in his full regalia. Music and rhythmic movement lend their aid in creating an appropriate atmosphere for healing

Facing page below. Sand painting of the Holy People of Hail Chant. Black Rain Boy and his sister, Blue Rain Girl, are walking around a lake. Four sacred plants – corn, beans, squash and tobacco – are placed diagonally, their roots extending into the lake. The boy carries lightning and sun-ray in his hands and travels on black and white lightning; the girl carries rain rope and sun-ray and travels on rainbows

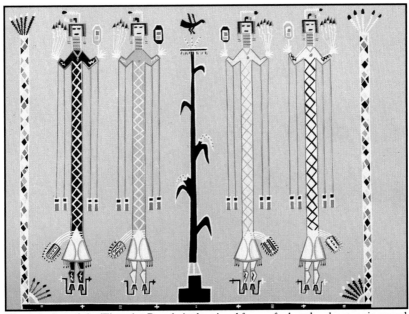

The painting of the Thunder People is the visual form of what the chanter sings and the dancers act. In the above painting the four long thin figures are Black, Blue, Yellow and White Thunder, the zigzags on their bodies are lightning. In one hand they hold octagonal hailstones, in the other lightning. They are standing, or travelling, on black and white lightning

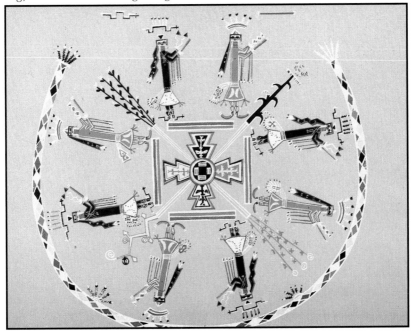

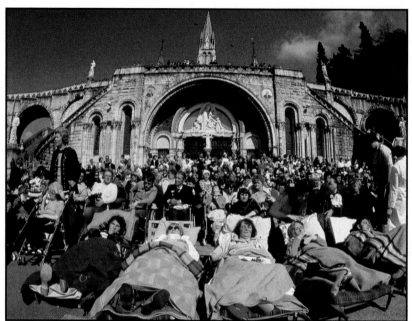

Pilgrims at Lourdes, those who are ill and the healthy who travel with them, wait for Mass in the Grotto to receive the healing blessings of the Virgin Mary

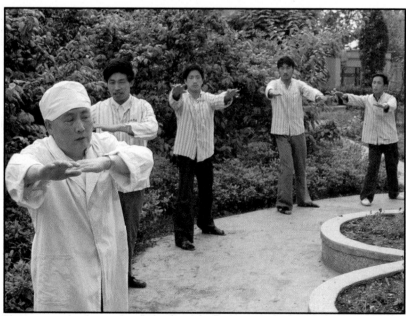

Qi gong can also be used to help the sick. Patients at the hospital are taught the movements by a traditional doctor who is a master of the art. He not only helps the patients to increase their *qi* but, in a Chinese version of healing by touch, he also passes his own *qi* directly into patients by touching acupuncture points

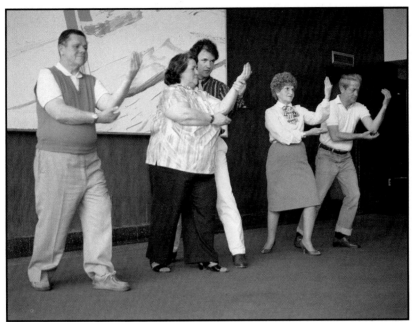

Patients at Boston's Lemuel Shattuck hospital learn to change bad habits of posture, movement and breathing developed over a lifetime

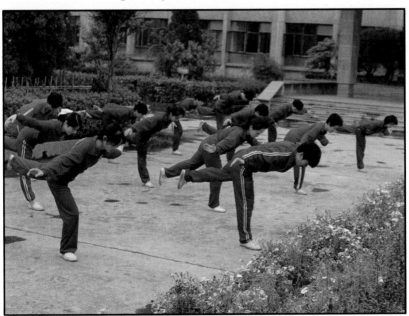

In China, the almost secret skills of *qi gong* are beginning to be taught widely. These students at the College of Traditional Medicine in Chengdu are practising the 'Flying Crane' sequence. These ancient exercises are designed to increase the internal energy, or *qi*, of the practitioners

127

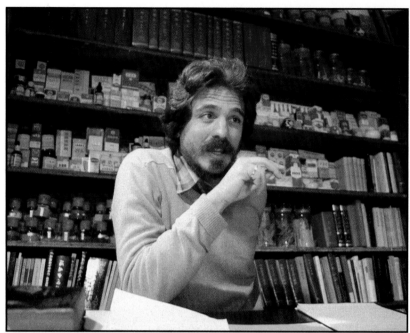

Ted Kaptchuk in his own consultation room

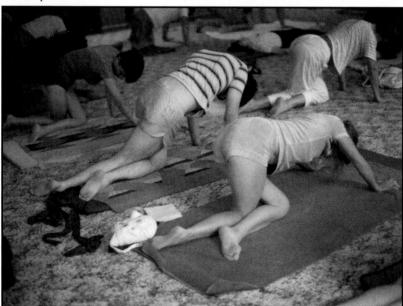

A Feldenkrais class for advanced students held in Toronto. Each lesson develops a pattern of movements that teach the body something more about its unused capabilities. Neither athleticism nor skill in performance are needed in these movements, whose purpose is focused on relating the brain to the body

share their world. They gain new insights from others who 'know', and even teach what they have learned.

Since I don't perform any specific therapy in the clinic, being, with Michael Zucker, the neutral co-ordinator, when I meet patients I offer them the freedom to take me to the important places in their lives. I let them set the pace. If they don't start a conversation, I usually ask what they like to do on a Sunday afternoon. Or what the best time in their life was. Or whether their illness taught them anything positive. They invariably share with me information about themselves that was never discussed in the clinic before. And they tell me how to repair a foreign car, how to make *lasagne*, what the grandchildren are up to, how it feels to carry a sack of groceries up the stairs with a bad back, and why they write poetry, the latest sample of which they will bring next time.

And the discussion can continue. We create a space where the patient can find his or her own place. Together, we rest from the anxious search for a cure and encounter each other's humanity. The discussion can deepen to where the pain can be shared – no longer just something to scramble away from but an experience of our common dilemma. The pain pushes us beyond childlike illusions of painlessness or wholeness. Pain and illness becomes a boundary existing because of our own aversion. Shirking the border creates a prison; meeting it is an encounter with fate, possibly a step to wisdom. These discussions can make the pain worse at first but then it becomes much easier to bear. Often a mutual bittersweet recognition and silence tells me to let the discussion rest.

Each one of our therapies has blind spots. During the team meeting, it is obvious that each discipline asks questions based on its picture of what is important. None can claim to know the patient exclusively. Only the psychiatrist asks about relationships to mothers and fathers; only the social worker asks about income and work; whereas the acupuncturist alone thinks it's important how many sweaters are worn or what the pulse at the radial artery feels like. These differences of opinions have to be smoothed out. Patients cannot receive every therapy. Is yoga better than *tai chi*? Is hypnotism more effective than biofeedback? Will individual psychotherapy undercut the meditation? What should be done when the acupuncturist disagrees with the nutritionist about diet? Only the strongest of practitioners can work in such a humbling environment.

Still when our practitioners complete their training they always recommend that others apply. The clinic does something special they say. By having their blind spots explicitly exposed on a daily basis, questions are raised and they are forced to their limits. They are forced to connect with that difficult-to-articulate evocative chord that lies hidden in every healing art. They learn to move from the facts of their training to what is unique, non-replicable and ineffable in their patient. The technicians of a particular medicine are transformed into healers who use a particular medicine.

And yet the healing performed at our clinic is more than the sum of the evaluations and treatments, more than the techniques and manipulations, even more than the skill and artistry of our staff. Each time a new patient arrives, I know that he or she will find one person on the staff (surprisingly it does not tend to be the same person) with whom they share something special. It is an exchange of trust, responsibility, reliance and caring that allows a patient to go through the healing process. We don't enjoy many of these kinds of relationships in life. The healer shares a painful, terrifying, fragile and dangerous time in our life. Aristotle defined it for the Western world when he wrote that the healer is a special friend because he 'shares your pleasure in what is good and your pain in what is unpleasant for your own sake'. This bond forms the foundation of the healing arts.

This is our open clinic. We are old enough as an institution to know that we are helping people; our evaluation studies confirm that. In the most recent pain performance examination, 70 per cent of our patients scored dramatic reduction of pain on the various tests. Sometimes a patient answers the questionnaires in a way that would indicate the pain is 'worse' on the 'objective scores'. I began an apologetic conversation with one such woman. She didn't understand my tone of voice. She told me she had learned how to cope with pain, to take care of herself, and that even in pain she could be a person. She had a new commitment to life and had changed from a victimised piece of protoplasm to a volunteer at a Save the Whales ecology centre. Our test counted her a failure; but she knew otherwise.

Recently we have expanded our research work. We want to continue adding to the fund of knowledge so important in our scientific culture. We acknowledge the opportunity that science has given us to do work hitherto unapproached, and probably only attemptable in the developed West.

Michael Croucher and I met after going to the East, for different reasons, some years ago. There we learnt to look with fresh eyes at the scientific medical approach, and so we gained, ironically, a new respect for modern medicine by getting away from it.

Let us now each tell our personal story of how we arrived at the 'open clinic'. For I see this concept as something that exists well beyond the Pain and Stress Relief Clinic in Boston. It exists wherever patients like Michael have the courage and self-knowledge to explore the healing arts.

I identify my life's work, in some ways, with the story of Lévi-Strauss' shaman, to which I have already alluded. This sceptic immersed himself in the medical lore of the Eskimos in order to expose what he thought to be the quackery of shamanism. He learned about massage, Arctic herbal lore, and even simple surgery, but most importantly he learned how to go into trance states, how to appease the insulted spirits of the walrus and the polar bear. He studied the dance that 'blows away' possession. He spat out pebbles, feathers and blood to rid the body of sickness, threw his voice across rooms to communicate with demons, and transferred sickness from humans into expendable objects such as sticks or dogs. He began to believe he could affect the minds, feelings and wills of people, even transplant their souls, giving them new names and genders. He could think with his entire body. Soon he felt he was living in the myths of his people and not in his own body. He was besieged for help by patients. Other shamans begged him to reveal his secrets. How much happier he would have been, he thought, if this Eskimo medicine were just the empty myth he had intended to expose. Instead, it kept working!

The story ends there. We don't know if this most famous of the shamans came to despise his hypocrisy or turned his understanding of the power of ritual into wisdom. I have felt a kindred spirit in the shaman. I know his tension well of being both comfortable and uncomfortable in several worlds. I turned from the study of oriental philosophy in an American university to its branch in a Chinese medical school. If Eastern thought had validity, I reasoned, it must show up in practice. Could this medicine of herbs and acupuncture stand up to the tests of real illness and disease? With that Western rite of passage, my degree, behind me, and bolstered by the restless, youthful enthusiasm for adventure, I set out to learn the medicine of the Far East.

In San Francisco I learned from Dr Hong that one painful elbow was 'wind' and another 'dampness'. They looked the same to me; it didn't make sense. This kind of apprenticeship was too slow for me after years of intellectual freedom and enquiry at a university. I knew I had to go farther west to reach the East. But I was told that it wouldn't be easy in China, where I would have to learn the language along with taking the medical courses. I plunged in anyway, finding a school willing to take me in Macao, near Hong Kong.

The Cultural Revolution of Mao Tse-tung was still going on at this time in mainland China. Accordingly, Chinese students from the surrounding countries of Indonesia, Burma, Thailand or Vietnam had to look elsewhere if they wanted to learn traditional Chinese medicine. These were my classmates, and both they and the Chinese teachers, most of whom came from the mainland, were suspicious of the American in their midst. In their countries, the traditional medicine was low-class compared to the high-tech, glamorous science of the West. Was I an agent for the CIA, a dropout, a Buddhist, a member of a splinter Maoist faction, or just a freak?

Slowly I was transformed from a Brooklyn Jew into a white-faced Chinese. From total rejection and mocking disparagement I moved to acceptance and finally friendship. My classmates appreciated the irony that someone coming from my university background was expected to ask thoughtful questions – it was the highest compliment for the teachers – whereas they had to listen in respectful silence. So they passed notes to me when they wanted questions asked. Gradually I forgot the prophet Jeremiah's passion for directness and truth and adopted the polite manner of an Oriental. After a crash course in Chinese I began to understand the lectures, learning to write in pictures instead of words. Rice replaced bread, while sticks and bowls replaced forks and spoons.

All this was accelerated by my being adopted into a Chinese family. My Chinese godmother had no heirs, so it fell upon me to perform the rites of worshipping the proper ancestors and spirits at such times as New Year and Grave Sweeping Day. I learned how to address aunts and uncles correctly, how to cook and clean. Inexorably I became part of the family, experiencing its sorrows and the creative energy of its joy. Their past trials through war and revolution became my history. I became adept at the rites of the Guan-Yin Buddhist cult. I could arrange the altar, calculate feast and fast days and taboo days, and celebrate the birthdays of such luminaries of the spirit world as the Jade Emperor and his heavenly court. To this day I can remember the power of that faith and I still fulfil my promise to perform the ritual for departed ancestors.

But to replace my world of medicine in some ways proved more difficult. I had expected to study such things as heart disease, hepatitis and haemophilia as something to be treated with 'natural' herbs, acupuncture, diet and exercise. Instead, this Western point of view was relegated to a secondary role, while the traditional notions of dampness and wind, *yin* and *yang* formed the main focus of attention. The subject might be a practical one such as insomnia or urination, but it was approached from the Chinese relationship with the entire environment and cosmos.

I'm not sure when I finally became at home in China and felt comfortable with Chinese medicine, but it may have been the day I listened to my godmother talk about the stroke her husband had suffered. She spoke of the 'wind' that was part of his illness. I saw him through her eyes and gripping language. Maybe I felt at one with China when the time came to bury my godfather and I took his soul through the rites of passage of the Chinese heavenly world. Maybe it was the day in clinic when I first saw *yin* and *yang* beyond the mere memorisation of lists of words; like the colour of someone's shirt, I could see wind and dampness. I was now ready to use Chinese medicine to treat the sick and heal the afflicted.

Even so, during her husband's illness I had turned my eyes away from a lesson about a different type of Chinese medicine which I wasn't prepared to see. My godmother had been ill, too. It was serious, and she had gone to a Western-style hospital for tumours in Canton for a diagnosis with X-rays and biopsies. It was thyroid cancer and chemotherapy was not yet available. She was told it was incurable, and my teachers of traditional Chinese medicine agreed. But she was mainly concerned about who would nurse her ailing husband. A devout soul, she went to consult the 'medicine Buddha'. This was one of the 'alternative' medicines of China – an ancient folk practice descended from earlier shamanic rites. She lit incense and candles to invoke the gods; she bowed, prayed, prostrated herself and cried. Finally she took some joss sticks and threw them: they came out to the number 146. The priest looked the number up in his huge, worn, dusty book, and told my godmother to drink one cup of tea brewed from the plums of a special tree for four weeks, and chant mantras all the while. Four weeks later the tumour was gone.

I would see years later, after returning to the United States, that Chinese medicine contained wheels within wheels, and that the traditional one that I had studied was far from the whole art of healing. I could have remained an acupuncturist and herbalist, set up a practice anywhere in the country, and ridden the crest of the wave of popularity of this alternative to scientific medicine. But I was driven to explore additional medical approaches. I began to pay attention to the cacophony of competing healing arts. It seemed that each system saw things that would be missed by others. What was background or irrelevant information for one practitioner would be pivotal for the next. Each somehow captured a different image in his conceptual camera. Each vision had a power – and each had blind spots. Many things were going on in the world, even in China, that my Chinese education missed, did not consider important or ignored. All the medical paradigms contained portions of truth; none was 'proven'. Medicine is the application of what people think is true about the cosmos to what is experienced in everyday life. In short I began to see what was to be the central theme of our Pain and Stress Relief Clinic: that the competition between medicines is not to prove that one or other of them is right. The reality of the person and his suffering is too large for any one medicine ever to comprehend.

The open clinic in the largest sense does not exist in any hospital, but in the range of practices presently scattered without any unifying programme throughout the world. We have seen how every speciality from acupuncture to osteopathy is now available in or near major population centres of the West. But it is rare in our society for a person to be introduced to one of these medicines without an experienced guide. Michael Croucher had that opportunity, and here is his story to parallel mine.

I can point to the exact moment in my life when I began to think about medicine in a way that has led to changes in the way I live, and to the writing of this book. It was in the city of Taipei, the capital of Taiwan, on 28 December 1982, where I was to meet a master of the soft Chinese martial art of *tai chi* to try to persuade him to take part in a documentary. I left the modern business centre and entered the old town where the streets are narrow and full of the vitality of Chinese life. I arrived at Master Hung's door, and from inside came a groan. The interpreter said, 'Master Hung mend broken bone.' We were waved in, and saw the master massaging oil into a young man's swollen, not broken, knee – an accident of training. It is normal for masters of martial arts to practise medicine in the East.

A small motorbike pulled up to the open door. Riding pillion was a small boy of eight or nine, clinging to his father and pressing an envelope tightly against his back. It contained an X-ray, which was immediately passed to the master. Space was somehow made for the father and son, and Master Hung removed a pile of old books from his X-ray viewer and switched it on. It was a badly broken elbow: fragments of bone could easily be seen on the viewer. This was my first surprise: here in an advanced city with several modern hospitals a severe injury was brought to a man with only a viewer, but the fact that Master Hung had one implied that it was frequently used.

Now the master turned his attention to the elbow, and the boy squirmed in pain on his father's knee as the large, powerful hands examined the break. Then I had my second surprise: the boy was sent back to the hospital on the bike, but only for another X-ray. I'd been told that the Chinese are the most practical people in the world, but here they were deliberately rejecting the obvious benefits of anaesthesia and the glamour of Western technology. Master Hung understood my concern; he explained that if surgery was not needed the bone would heal faster if set the Chinese way. What about the boy's evident pain? He would have to wait several hours for an anaesthetic at the hospital, I was told patiently; this way, he would be in his own world and would be comfortable very soon. There was yet a third X-ray when the second showed a bone still out of place, and now the splinting could begin.

This was my third surprise: the master was using thin pieces of bamboo instead of plaster. As he worked, he told me through the interpreter that he had used no drugs because this way the boy would have to recover only from shock. But the bamboo? No, plaster hides the injury, he said, and it should be massaged daily. Rigid, the bone heals slowly and the muscles atrophy. It seemed unlikely to me, but I didn't realise then that bamboo has astonishing strength, nor could I know that in 1984 scientific research would show that it is often better to splint bones than to put them in plaster, for exactly the reasons that Master Hung had given.

With the boy now sitting proudly on his knee, the master took time to tell me about Chinese medicine. He practised as a doctor, mainly with acupuncture, as well as in bone-setting and manipulation. No, he said, acupuncture would not have been useful to relieve pain here. This was a distortion of its main purpose, which is in chronic conditions. Instead, while he was working on the boy he had pressed points to relieve shock and pain. The type of acupuncture sensationalised by the Western media, as an alternative to anaesthesia in operations, required hours of preparation.

During the months of research and filming of my documentary on the masters of martial arts I was often similarly taken aback. Each master taught me something different. I could not remain a dispassionate observer as the new picture of therapy took shape in my mind. This culture had to be respected, for in its antiquity and perhaps wisdom it had served a population far outnumbering any other in the world.

My mind had been opened, as well, to those healing arts I had ignored in my own culture as being 'alternative', which is to say subordinate, if not downright outlandish. And I was also drawn to that arena of healing where my thinking would converge with the conception that Ted Kaptchuk has of this process: magic.

Near Tokyo lives a master who teaches the refined art of using the Japanese sword in the same way that it has been taught at his school since the fourteenth century; he may well be the world's greatest master of the sword. A form of Buddhism, 'Esoteric', originally used to prepare warriors for battle, is now taught here to advanced students. More to my purpose, this ritual is also used in healing. Visualise the scene. The master sits among his patients, drawing on paper complex symbols and diagrams of the human body showing where their illness is centred. Each piece of paper is folded into the shape of a fan and clipped to a piece of bamboo. Placing them on an altar, he prays before them, forming mantras with interlocking patterns of his fingers. The master then strokes the centre of illness of each patient and bids them to take the fans to a riverbank, to be left there without looking back. I later observed one arthritic woman, who could scarcely bend her knees on arrival, walking away freely down the steps. The master would only claim that his patients generally left cheerful, with at least temporary relief.

As the filming of the documentaries progressed I was confronted with one cultural splinter after another from the past, often several within the same country. On an island off the coast of Japan, some 400 miles south of Tokyo, I met a master of the fighting art of Shorinji Kempo who was renowned for his skills as a manipulator. Master Bando demonstrated for my benefit his special technique for reviving a person who had been knocked out, for example, in sports. In India I watched Ayurvedic doctors practise the neglected martial art of kalaripayit. In addition to deep massage by the feet and manipulation, their range of techniques included the prescription of a mantra and restrictions of such things as cardamom seeds. I watched one of these practitioners heal a badly infected, swollen leg with herbs and massage when it seemed to be in desperate need of an antibiotic.

My conversion to a broader view of medicine would not have been complete without a painful personal experience in Hong Kong. Two days before I was due to fly home with my family, I lifted my two-year-old daughter and, as often happens when one least expects it, strained my back. I crawled into a taxi which took me across Hong Kong to Master Chan, the Kung Fu practitioner whom I had filmed that week. I staggered past the watch-seller's booth, the travel agency, the tailor's cutting table and the Kung Fu exercise hall like a man pretending to ride a motorbike. With a not very inscrutable smile on his face he examined me in front of his friends, who took the opportunity to gossip openly about the follies of the West. At last he stretched out his finger and with exquisite precision placed it on the centre of the trouble on my bare back. Then he rubbed in a cream of his own making, massaged my back and applied a hot poultice. He had told me of the forty herbs that went into it, and of even more complicated mixtures, especially the one used for knitting bones. And he had warned me of the dangers of leaving any bruise untreated, which we routinely do in the West. The Chinese believe that any untreated bruise is a site for future trouble.

Home safely and mending, I decided to test what I had been filming. I went to a famous English acupuncturist even though I felt healthy. My only complaint was a tendency to migraines. He did the things I had witnessed on my tour, felt my pulse, examined my tongue and listened intently to what I thought were routine answers. Then he advised me that my kidney and liver meridians were out of balance; he would harmonise them. The needles were inserted in various places over my body; they were not painless but easily bearable for my half-hour on the couch. I noticed a tendency in the next few days to drink more water, and to get rid of it more often. And after three weeks I noted a thin film of dust on my aspirin bottle.

I have not become a 'born again' devotee of complementary medicines, but I have learned to experiment with my health care. On my next visit to the acupuncturist, I was advised to have my neck and back looked at by an osteopath. And I have now signed up my children for visits to a homeopath.

I think I can speak frankly about the inherent problems of competing medical systems. There is a tendency for each to become evangelistic and unobjective, to see the whole of healing as their preserve, and to denigrate other approaches – all because of the subtle effects of the marketplace. As with Ted, however, for me the positive side of these systems looms large where the edges of our drug-oriented medicine seem withdrawn. In particular, I would now like to explore, from the point of view of the well-informed patient, the neglected arts of moving and eating that engage us for most of our waking hours.

9·THE·LOST·ART· OF·MOVING

At about the turn of the century, two ominous but almost unnoticed social changes began to take shape in the Western developed nations. The food supply became more and more degraded with the advent of large-scale processing, and simultaneously physical labour started to become increasingly unnecessary for large numbers of people in the home or the workplace. There were prophets who warned about the inevitable demise in personal health that these changes would bring. But the coming of vaccines and, later, antibiotics tended to mask these dangers with optimistic analyses of life expectancy – which go on, incidentally, to this day. John Powles describes a parallel development in the medical profession: 'The germ theory of disease came just in time to save the faltering public prestige of doctors.'

When attention was finally focused on poor diets and lack of exercise, it came as a sort of rearguard concession from the ascendant medical world. Nutrition, which will be covered in Chapter 10, was granted only a preventative role. And even now exercise is scribbled into a prescription in a generalised, which is to say trivialised, way. It is assumed that any form of exercise will do. I intend to treat it here, however, as truly a healing art, and one with many specific uses.

I can make this point quite clearly in the case of that most ubiquitous of present-day exercise programmes, aerobics. Long-distance running, swimming, cycling and other sustained activities that raise the heartbeat to a range of about 120–140 are considered aerobic, which means requiring a continuous supply of air. Such activities as sprinting or tennis consume only short bursts of air. Aerobic exercise for at least thirty minutes a day, three times a week, has been correlated in many studies with decreased incidence of heart disease. We speak of aerobics as being preventive of heart attacks, as indeed it is statistically, yet its potential for healing is expressed in a number of ways. First, the above-mentioned aerobic programme is clearly correlated with an increase in HDL, or high-density lipoprotein,

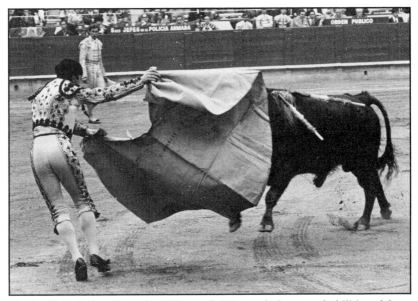

The bullfight is based on the different fighting techniques and abilities of four-legged animals and men. The matador, with great economy, sways and turns on his two feet. The bull charges with great force on his four feet but lacks the agility to follow the movements of the man

which can help retard atherosclerosis; second, it can discourage the bad habit of smoking, and is one of the least traumatic ways of doing so; third, it can stimulate better food choices by placing demands on the body for increased complex carbohydrates; fourth, it can stimulate the digestive process to correct intestinal disorders; and fifth, it can induce fuller use of the capillaries and hormonal systems that interlock in the body, to help pre-empt circulatory diseases and stress. The vitality and healthy glow that are the signs of a well-exercised body undoubtedly go hand in hand with improved mental functioning. Only the scientific underpinnings of this model are new, however; the spirit of this prescription can be traced back to the Greek ideal of a sound mind in a sound body.

So much has been written about popular sports that the examples quoted here are quite sufficient to illustrate the general health benefits of exercise. In the enthusiasm for aerobics, however, the exercise of the entire body has either been neglected or reduced to the purpose of losing weight and gaining a better figure. I would like to concentrate, therefore, on those arts of movement that deserve wider attention and can contribute to improvements throughout our person.

The way that our skeleton, with its covering of muscles and

ligaments, has developed is a triumph of engineering. Some would claim otherwise; and I agree that for the purpose of standing still for long hours on production lines or slouching in front of television sets the body is badly designed. You do not see bad posture in animals. But man has the ability to subject himself to discomfort by making his actions conform to his brain. The fact that man evolved to be superior to all the animals on the African plains tells us a lot about the potential enemy to our bodies that we all carry around in our skulls.

This simple observation lies at the root of many of the corrective therapies of bodily movement I would like to explore. In our evolution from some kind of tree-climbing animal, we developed a special skill to which we give little thought. Other animals can look behind them, and often must in order to survive. But only man can turn easily, without wasting energy; turning around his centre of gravity which is located four-fingers width below the navel and quite close to the spine. We need only to move our feet and we are poised, facing the other direction, ready to run, to dodge or to fight. The body of an animal is fixed by the planting of his legs, and to turn they have to use large amounts of energy to shift their mass around. A simple experiment shows this. Hold a metal bar at one end between the fingers. A tiny effort will spin it. Then lay it down and spin it around its middle. The work needed to achieve this is many times greater. Taken to its extreme, this characteristic of man is beautifully exhibited in the ballet dancer spinning across a stage or a skater adjusting the speed of spin by changing the stretch of the arms.

The mere ability to keep one's balance, to which we give little thought except on a lurching bus or train, is not uniquely human by any means but is unimaginably complex in our upright body. By looking into balance a little more closely, we will be able to appreciate the puzzle of back problems, tension, and even some joint pains that we usually assume to be due, like disease, to an outside invader.

As soon as a baby has enough strength, it will hold its head poised, opposing by means of the counter-tension of the supporting muscles the gravitational pull that occurs with the slightest change of its position in its mother's arms. So the baby learns balance from its head downwards – the most necessary and the most difficult feat first, since at birth the head constitutes about two-fifths of the entire body weight. As the growing child goes through the various phases of crawling, sitting, standing, walking and running, the organs of balance in the inner ear adjust each new set of muscles that come into play. The poise of the body is fluid from moment to moment in this

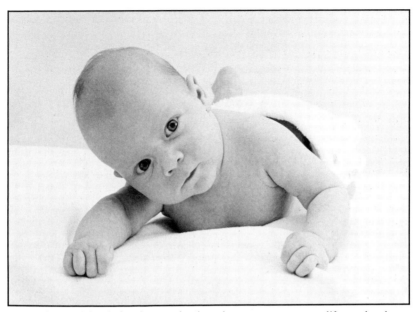

We are born with a balancing mechanism that means we try to lift our head to a vertical position which keeps the eyes horizontal

animal-like, natural growth. Only later do we begin to distort this sense of balance by consciously adjusting to the various postures of standing in lines, playing the violin, or bending over patients all day in a dentist's surgery. We fall from a free-form ideal into rigid, artificially learned postures. Unlike the developing baby, we stop exploring new twists and turns, new hops and skips. Fixed in habitual patterns of movement, unwilling to extend ourselves much beyond them, we subject our bodies, and perhaps our minds, to an assortment of ailments attributed to accidents or microbes or even old age. Our practitioners then treat these locally, to little avail.

So oblivious are we to our daily contortions to maintain our balance that all of this may sound far-fetched, so we should look further into the complex mechanisms involved. Suppose we try to make a model of a person, starting from the feet. To make the wobbling bones of the leg stand on them at all we would have to attach pieces of elastic to them. If we can get beyond the knee to the pelvis by the same tactic, we have to establish a sort of platform there on which to anchor the spine. Then we must somehow balance the pull of the muscles on both sides and the unpredictable weight of the internal organs stacked on top of the pelvis. Then there is the pile of ribs, breastbone and shoulder bones supporting the neck, all of

141

which ultimately is designed to carry the head. This swaying tower would represent a big enough challenge to construct for a single position. But human beings move constantly, even in sleep. (If you have ever suffered from a pulled medial collateral ligament in the knee you will know that any so-called position of rest cannot balance the knee without sleep-disturbing pain.) Even at its most relaxed, the body is constantly adjusting its muscular tensions.

We can now see why the advocates of a number of theories of movement put such emphasis on the idea of use. A story is often told of how Jim Thorpe, an American Olympic athlete, took part in an exercise experiment with babies in the early 1920s. When asked to duplicate or mimic the movements of a two-year-old over the course of a day, he was unable to keep up! In the normal course of growing up and going to work we fall into patterns of movement which in themselves may not be harmful but which preclude everything else.

Necessary though aerobic exercise may be, therefore, without a greater range of movement the running or swimming that this entails may only add years to our life and not life to our years. Narrowly repetitive exercise routines may in fact create new fixed patterns instead of expanding our possibilities. In the initial enthusiasm of starting an aerobic programme, we may also fail to heed the warning signs of stress, try to 'run through pain', or attempt to short-cut the procedure by failing to stretch, warm up and cool down. We may also take the act of breathing too much for granted; a simple rule of thumb in aerobics is to be able to maintain a conversation or be able to sing while exercising the lungs and heart.

Closer to a well-rounded exercise programme are those sports which also involve thought processes. There are meditative aspects to long-distance running, and hunting game and the strategy of football present opportunities for a fuller range of faculties to come into play. Yet even the most demanding sports are self-limiting, and so we look for ways of supplementing them.

In this search, I would like to emphasise the mental aspect along with the ideal of total use of the body. Some thinking is, of course, automatic, as in riding a bicycle even after long years of not doing it. When we first tried to learn as children, thinking about it helped very little – just as it fails us when we first take up skiing, hitting a golf ball or hang-gliding. But once the pattern has been made in our brain, our balance mechanism stretches to accommodate this new knowledge and it is never forgotten. In the best of the modern exercise gyms, little thinking is required except of the automatic kind. The range of workouts is, nevertheless, quite impressive. Exercises seldom attempted are suggested by a wide array of equipment. The biochemical theories on which this machinery is based are quite elaborate, taking into account new developments in kinesiology and body-building. The gym is a good start towards a well-rounded and properly modulated programme.

Some attempt has been made to introduce thinking, or at least aerobic benefits, into 'pumping iron'. In so-called 'circuit' weight training, participants move quickly from station to station to maintain an elevated pulse. The epitome of such a programme is the popular, outdoor 'parcourse' system found in many cities in the United States. Something like an aerobic golf course, or an advanced playground, this carefully laid-out exercise tour offers a complete range of movement and standards to aim for. Yet critics point out that aerobics only works its benefits if the *same* muscle group is involved for a twenty- to thirty-minute period. It is this extended workout that makes muscle cells more efficient in extracting oxygen from the blood, thereby placing less of a demand on the heart to pump blood. As any consistent runner knows, a lowered resting heart rate is the first signal of aerobic success.

Some exercise may, in fact, be counter-productive as far as the heart is concerned. Isometric contractions, for example, pressing the palms of the hands together and pressing as hard as you can repeatedly, tense the muscles without moving them; this sort of tension inhibits the flow of blood in those muscles and so raises blood pressure. It is therefore more beneficial to the heart, if not the size of the muscles, to concentrate on frequent repetitions with less load. In short, the best guidelines are endurance and variety, as offered by modern dance, 'jazzercise' and yoga.

But before looking at that fascinating world of what I term 'thoughtful movement', I must emphasise how much we take for granted in what is called 'muscle sense'. Just as we rarely give a thought to the staggering demands of balance, so we consider this sixth sense to be scientific exaggeration. Properly known as proprioception or sense of oneself, not only is this faculty critical to our sense of wellbeing, it is intrinsic to our ego. Here indeed is the issue of mind and body joined, and an avenue of the healing process opened.

A single case, dramatically told by a rather unusual patient, recently brought this sixth sense to public attention. Dr Oliver Sacks is a London-born professor of neurology at Albert Einstein College of Medicine in New York. In his 1985 book, *A Leg to Stand On*, he recounts the story of a hiking injury that left him with a surgically attached leg in which he had no feeling at all. This was more than the familiar feeling of numbness: the leg was alien to him.

> . . . I gazed at it, and felt I don't know you, you're not part of me, and, further, I don't know this 'thing', it's not part of anything. *I had lost my leg.* . . . I was now an amputee, but not an ordinary amputee. For the leg, objectively, externally, was still there, it had disappeared subjectively, internally. . . . I had lost the inner image, or representation, of the leg.

Noting the irony of another patient with no leg and yet all the feelings of one – a common sensation among genuine amputees – Dr Sacks began a long process of recovery that led to a theory of therapeutics. First there are some involuntary twitches in the 'thing', then he is able to swing it like some limb of a ventriloquist's doll. Like an adult trying a bicycle for the first time, he tries to teach himself what should be spontaneous. Finally, as Dr Daniel X. Freedman describes it, 'The return of command, of uncalculated certainty, an "I", arrives in one swoop of unsummoned "grace" manifest in sheer action.' Using the recovery of sensation and motion in his leg as an extreme case, Dr Sacks constructed a model of the healing process. First, healing consists of many events, often discontinuous. Secondly, an intermediary is necessary – a third party, a healer. Finally, action is the force needed for breaking the log-jams in the river of health. An unexpected push into a swimming pool triggered Dr Sacks' full recovery, as his love of swimming suddenly took him off guard.

Ideas from various cultures begin to converge. The Zen master also employs the surprise factor to evoke responses from the centre of the person. Dr Sacks borrowed the concept of 'centring' the patient from other touchstones. His friend, the poet W. H. Auden, suggested music as a good device for summoning the 'I' in a patient. 'A living personal center' is how he describes it – and it correlates with the idea of intactness that is at the core of my idea of coming to grips with illness.

With this background it is easier to see a rationale for the movement and manipulation arts of otherwise dubious-sounding therapies. Let's look more closely at such techniques as *qi gong, tai chi*, the Alexander Method and the teachings of Moshe Feldenkrais. It is probably helpful to suspend judgement at this point, to immerse yourself uncritically in each culture, with the purpose of achieving a point of view without reference to your own. In short, at this stage it is more important to understand than to evaluate.

In the Far East the links between the martial arts and healing are very strong, unlikely though this may seem. There is a practical side to this: in Hong Kong, masters of kung fu finance their classes by treating bruises, broken bones and painful backs. In Okinawa, masters of karate work on patients with shiatsu massage. In southern India, masters of kalaripayit conduct their classes in the morning and evening, practising Ayurvedic medicine in between. But there is more than a financial relationship. A martial art is thought to stimulate that internal flow of energy which the Chinese call *chi* and the Indians *prana*. It is this that brings the crowds out before dawn to perform the stately *tai chi* exercises in the parks of the major cities of China, for this is when *chi* is flowing strongly through nature. Only a person who has *chi* under control is considered capable of fighting, but that is only part of the picture. The balance of the forces of nature, which we have seen as a primary concept in various ancient medical systems, is also considered to be the rationale for practising the martial arts.

Undoubtedly the exercise system with a philosophical dimension best known to the West is yoga. In its fullest sense yoga is a way of life, but it appeals to Westerners at the simple level of relaxed, controlled stretching and breathing. In an interesting Foreword to B. K. S. Iyengar's *Light on Yoga*, the musician Yehudi Menuhin captures the essence of the Eastern point of view:

> The practise of Yoga induces a primary sense of measure and proportion. Reduced to our own body, our first instrument, we learn to play it, drawing from it maximum resonance and harmony. With unflagging patience we refine and animate every cell as we return daily to the attack, unlocking and liberating capacities otherwise condemned to frustration and death. . . . By its very nature it is inextricably associated with universal laws: for respect for life, truth, and patience are all indispensable factors in the drawing of a quiet breath, in calmness of mind and firmness of will. . . . No mechanical repetition is involved and no lip service as in the case of good resolutions or formal prayers. By its very nature it is each time and every moment a living act. . . .

Although this spiritual vision of yoga is broadly understood in the West, its healing potential for such maladies as headaches, backaches, varicose veins or digestive problems is rarely considered. In India, various postures or *asanas* are used for a whole array of diseases or discomforts that we would deal with surgically or at least with drugs. But these postures, which seem impossible or painful at first, are not intended as instant answers. In learning yoga positions one simultaneously trains the entire neurological and immunological network. As we have seen, yoga-like methods are now routinely employed at major hospitals to induce the 'relaxation response'. It is as if two work parties have been burrowing into a mountain from opposite sides: from the West come disease crews and from the East come meditation crews; they converge on the idea of stress.

The Chinese expression of exercise has similarities with the Indian one in its attempt to come to terms with nature rather than simply strengthen or relax the human body. From the earliest written record of Chinese exercise, by a doctor named Hua Tuo in the first or second century, we know that they were based on the movements of five animals: the deer, stork, tiger, bear and monkey. The ancient Taoists studied animals in great detail, with the idea not of mimicking them, but of learning their nature. Various movements were classified as aggressive or passive, the former naturally becoming the province of the martial arts as *tai chi*. But both sets of exercise were considered important to a fighter, to balance his internal strength and control *chi*, or force. The advanced levels of these exercises, attained after years of study, can be used specifically as healing arts.

Throughout the centuries the Chinese kept a form of exercise to themselves that is only now being opened up to the general public. Specifically a healing art, *qi gong* is alleged to have been the source of Chairman Mao's vigour and longevity. It is now out of the hands of private masters and in the hospitals, where it is used as a kind of physical therapy. At this level it has the same rationale as acupuncture or herbalism – to balance the forces of nature. At a second level it is practised by what we might call faith healers – masters who supposedly can focus their *chi* on an injury or disease location. Patients have reported heat flowing from a master's fingers and from them through the meridian of their bodies as *chi* flows from the master; *chi* that he has built up within himself by practising *qi gong*.

Throughout its history the West has remained remarkably innocent of the concept of movement as a healing art; only in the twentieth century have we developed any sort of organised programme or theory of exercise as a corrective. Two names are well known in this field: F. M. Alexander and Moshe Feldenkrais; in a sense, both men had something to say about posture as the source of many of our ills, but both were also restrained in their claims.

The Alexander Method was developed by an Australian actor, at about the turn of the century, for the specific purpose of helping to project the voice on stage. To this day one can spot a follower of the method by the way the actor's or actress's head is poised, but there is also a more general theory that has application to everyone from schoolchildren to the aged. The solution Alexander discovered to his immediate problem of voice projection is direct and understandable: actors assumed that the way to make their voices carry was to tilt the head backwards, but this action tended to compress the spine and vocal chords. In trying to overcome that tendency Alexander hit on a larger truth – that years of misuse or disuse cannot easily be overcome. He phrased this broadly in the axiom that is central to his theory: use determines function. The muscles that support the head have to be *used* in a new way to allow the vocal chords to function properly, and this concept applies to all the functions of the body. Taken to its conclusion, this theory implies that physical postures created by disuse lead to distinctive behavioural patterns.

This logical leap is suspect in our culture. A man cowers because he is afraid; his cowering does not cause the fear. Yet the case is not always this clear. Menuhin has this to say in *Light on Yoga*:

> The practise of Yoga over the last fifteen years has convinced me that most of our fundamental attitudes to life have their physical counterparts in the body. . . . Thwarted, warped people condemning the order of things, cripples criticising the upright, autocrats slumped in expectant coronary attitudes, the tragic spectacle of people working out their own imbalance and frustration on others.

Is is possible that our mental and emotional lives are crippled by habits of posture that subtly turn us into imitators of what we look like? There is a danger here of falling into the old fallacy of believing that there is a criminal physical type; but there is also much room for speculation about physical limitations distorting our larger lives.

Moshe Feldenkrais worked quite independently of Alexander, since they were not contemporaries, yet this Russian-born Israeli created a system of bodily retraining that is a logical culmination of the Australian's work. Feldenkrais had an unusual combination of talents, all of which contributed to the movement theory he postulated relatively late in life. As in Alexander's case, it was a personal problem that triggered his thinking. He had been a judo expert in the 1930s, when that sport was virtually unknown in the West; he had studied physiology in Paris, played football, and worked as a scientist in London during the Second World War. It was in this job that he slipped on the deck of a submarine and reinjured a knee – much like Dr Sacks. In recuperating, he found that he had to relearn how to walk in order to do it painlessly. From this experience came a remarkable book with the intriguing title *Body and Mature Behaviour: A Study of Anxiety, Sex, Gravitation, and Learning*.

147

Like many innovators, Feldenkrais was given to sweeping generalisations and grand formulations that make quotation difficult. Yet this and succeeding books, not to mention great clinical success, stamped him as one of the originals of our time. He described his general premise in these words:

> Unused parts of the body grow weak and atrophied; other parts bear a correspondingly heavier burden and are overworked; and the body becomes a caricature of the human frame . . . and a whole series of acts become excluded and impossible. Rationally, we convince ourselves that we do not really want . . . to perform such acts and they are totally withdrawn from our repertory of normal use.

Note the reference here to the 'enemy' we carry around with us: the brain. Human beings are unique in the animal kingdom in their ability to convince their bodies that something unnatural for them is what they should be doing.

When driving a car that pulls to one side on braking, one steers to compensate, and soon that adjustment to one's normal driving pattern becomes automatic. Similarly, we compensate for that most important part of the body, the head:

> When the head and pelvis are correctly held, all the range of their movements, and those of the rest of the body, are used, explored, or tried normally, without any special attention. When they are not, the attitude or posture can be likened to a groove into which the person sinks, never to leave unless some special force makes him do so. With time, the groove deepens . . . a person will resort to the most awkward and tiresome (to other people) procedures in turning the head, but will obstinately avoid lifting it into that position from which turning is normally easy.

Feldenkrais adds a striking parallel on the emotional plane: '. . . where the immature person uses detours, roundabout ways instead of direct, simple methods'.

A Feldenkrais teacher might demonstrate our physical limitations by asking us to scratch between our shoulder blades. Most of us give up trying to do this at some time in our lives. But if we are taught to move in some other way, we suddenly find we have required the flexibility to scratch our backs. In reaching for a book on a shelf slightly beyond arm's length, habit tells us to twist our shoulders to get it; but we can learn to stretch the entire arm, including the shoulder blade, just as naturally. The Feldenkrais idea is to re-educate the body to make fuller use of its capabilities.

Though Feldenkrais died in 1984 he left behind some intriguing tapes of sessions conducted by himself, which he called 'trainings'. It is here that his Socrates-like personality comes to the fore, drawing the student along so that he solves problems on his own. The point of a 'training' is seldom mentioned at the start; after an hour of fairly hard work the student finds himself achieving a level of movement that was unthinkable at the beginning. His jaw may become relaxed, or he may be able to raise his knee to touch his nose – all at the end of apparently irrelevant movements. It is somewhat eerie to see sixty or eighty students of all ages and builds moving on their bellies to the commands of a man who is no longer alive, examining themselves according to his suggestions, noticing the action of muscles and bones in some simple movement, monitoring their breathing and learning something as simple as how to lie down without assuming a tense position. Bodies get into habits even in sleep.

A full training session for possible teachers of Awareness Through Movement involves three or four one-hour classes a day for eight weeks. The individual spends the following year developing these exercises, then they return for another eight weeks. The complete course takes four sets of lessons. Feldenkrais insisted that this was simply re-education, not training for a specific purpose, such as flexibility. Because they involve intense mental concentration, the sessions are taxing; but the promise of effortless movement and attendant emotional and mental liveliness draws thousands of students to Feldenkrais practitioners throughout Europe, Israel, and America.

A second part of the Feldenkrais programme deals directly with what we would call healing and what he would insist is still a matter of reprogramming the brain. Functional Integration requires a trained practitioner, who uses manipulation, and often involves seriously ill or impaired patients. I participated in several sessions literally to get the feel for this aspect of Feldenkrais, and I observed some rather remarkable uses of the system in treatment. Even my brief experience with practitioners convinced me, far more than the theoretical framework in Feldenkrais' books, that there is indeed much to be learned here.

Even someone who has experienced a workout in yoga, massage or the more unusual movement therapies will still be quite surprised by their first Functional Integration session. The first impression is of naturalness and gentleness. There is no gym-like atmosphere; you remove your shoes, jacket and glasses, if you wear them, and lie down on a low table with a foam rubber pad under your knees. You are now asked to place yourself completely in the hands of the practitioner, and not to 'help' when he lifts your arm or leg. With a few deft probes of your legs, the teacher quickly achieves a relaxed state, in which a quieting pulse seems to course up your spine. The emphasis is on releasing tensions and reopening old blockages. After the first session you feel more confident and looser; in the second, third and fourth the feeling intensifies. There seems to be a quiet communication between the teacher and your muscles, ligaments and bones that has not happened before.

There is no suggestion of a 'quick fix'. Feldenkrais himself thought that one should have as many sessions as one's age. In this, as in his intense desire to explain the theory behind his methods, he is very much a part of Western scientific culture, just as *tai chi* springs from Chinese understanding of the cosmos. His most famous case history, the subject of his book *The Story of Nora*, is an object lesson in the scientific approach to medical treatment.

A middle-aged Parisian woman, the victim of a stroke that had left her unable to read or write or even dress herself, Nora had come to Feldenkrais, in Israel, as a last resort. She was unable to match her right foot with her right shoe; and she faced a life of disoriented dependency. There was nothing in the medical literature to suggest a starting point – except Feldenkrais' wide-ranging familiarity with the Swiss child psychologist Piaget, with the martial arts, and with the healing of his own knee. Painfully, patiently, he searched for the simplest accomplishment that Nora could achieve. He improvised, putting a straw in her mouth to help her move her eyes to the words on the page, drawing letters on her hands to help her recognise shapes. Each small triumph reinforced the complex structure of her achievement. Then they went on to new tasks. There was no pre-arranged theory or programme, only a way of thinking. As Nora returned to a normal life, it became clear that she was to relearn everything, like a child. In a bittersweet coda to the story, Nora and Feldenkrais met a few years later on Zurich railway station. Now fully confident and off on a shopping trip, she greeted him politely and then disappeared into the crowd.

My own observation of Feldenkrais practitioners corroborated Nora's story. In the early 1980s I visited a summer school in Rhode Island for young paraplegics, paralysed in varying degrees from spinal cord damage. The six-week session was itself organised by a paraplegic, to give a little more hope to others like him, as he put it, 'to fight back'. Among the techniques he had assembled were physiotherapy, Rolfing (a searching deep tissue massage), and Functional Integration, offered by a Feldenkrais teacher of long experience,

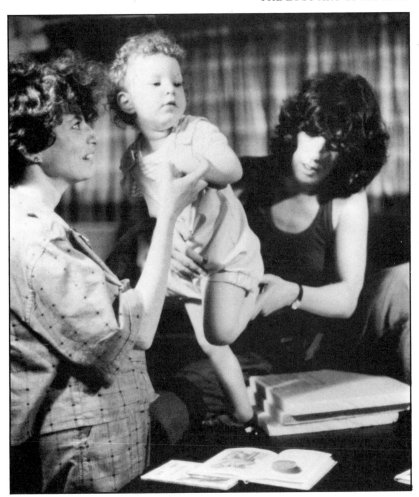

In the practice of Feldenkrais the relationship is always that of teacher and pupil. The teaching of this little brain-damaged girl is like a game, the Feldenkrais techniques concealed in laughter. Her mother also learns from Anat Baniel what her daughter can achieve and how to continue the effect of the lessons

Carl Ginsberg. Tragic victims of car crashes and other accidental misfortunes, the twenty or so young people I saw were achieving results that the medical profession regards as impossible.

One young man, told he would never walk again, was asked to search for the tiniest response. After many hour-long sessions he was able to stand upright and to raise his head. To him this minute improvement was a wonderful moment, because it implied the opportunity to move the muscles of his chest and back again, which in turn would lead to further advances. At the end of the six weeks he

151

was able to move under his own power with a single support.

To build from a twitch in the toe, to a sensation in the foot, and then perhaps some control of the foot and finally a spreading of sensation up the leg is almost a fairytale idea of medicine – and yet it is what healers such as Carl Ginsberg rely on. Another patient who stands out in my mind is an extraordinary example of this approach – a woman of thirty who had been immobilised for eighteen years after a road accident. She had felt some regeneration in her legs through a slight pain, but her doctor had told her that this was impossible. When she persisted in her claim she was sent to a psychiatrist, who also denied that she could feel pain. She began to lie to everyone about her feelings. She told me, 'I only feel whole when I'm asleep, so when I wake up I try to stay still as long as I can to keep that feeling of a whole body.' That very day she was able to move the big toe of her right foot for the first time in eighteen years. It was the culmination of six weeks at the school. 'It takes so long for the message to get down there,' she said.

I watched a six-year-old girl with cerebral palsy balance herself on her knees for the first time, supported only at the hips. She gave such a cry of joy at this sensation that no other medical corroboration was needed. This experience was all the more emotional for me since I had seen a tape of Feldenkrais working with her, virtually since birth, on eye and hand co-ordination. When he became ill, just before he died, Anat Baniel took over the child's case. While I watched, she taught her to stick out her tongue and touch her lips with it. One year later I filmed that child walking without support. It was another dramatic demonstration of the Feldenkrais concept that a damaged child has to be taught everything that a normal child would learn unconsciously in growing up. There are no short-cuts: no child can afford to miss any part of the learning process. If one never learns to crawl as a child, something will be missing as an adult.

From the appallingly difficult problems of handicapped children and from teachers like Feldenkrais, we may discover things about ourselves to which all our science has been blind. Exercise is more than burning up calories. Movement is more than stretching. The presence of a mind in our person, and all that this means from sensation to higher forms of reasoning, is paradoxically most obvious in the way our bodies move.

10·THE·LOST·ART· OF·EATING

There is a time-honoured and plausible theory about human nutrition, obvious to anyone who has observed animal behaviour: our own uncluttered taste buds are the surest guide to good eating habits. We lose the art of eating, according to this explanation, for much the same reason that we lose control of our movements. Through disuse and misuse at the earliest age, we neglect our full range of tastes, and that enemy within, the brain, allows us to compensate with foods that please us emotionally instead of nutritionally. For much of this we can blame the baby food manufacturers who reared us on sugar and salt, or the adult food manufacturers who removed nutrients and replaced them with substances to prolong their shelf life, but we were all born free. Why then do we over-eat, crave chocolate and 'white food' that requires little chewing, and mistake the fat-laden products of fast-food emporia for a hearty meal? Before looking at the evidence for our present malnutrition in the midst of abundance, we must consider the evolution of our eating habits – how, in brief, we have become separated from natural patterns of feeding in spite of, or because of, our status as kings of the animal world. Some sixty-five years ago, Dr Leonard Williams had this to say as the conclusion to the first entry under the word 'vitamines', as it was then spelt, in one of the early editions of *Encyclopedia Britannica*:

> The discovery of the vitamines presents would-be scientists with a much needed lesson in humility. It reminds us that, in evolving man, Nature provided him with the foods necessary to his growth, development, and well-being, and that in interfering with those natural foods by cooking, sterilising, and refining, he has sacrificed their efficacy, sometimes to his greed, but more to his arrogant assumption of superior knowledge, with the result that he has not only promoted the prevalence of preventable disease, but has actually created others which but for his misdirected energy would have had no existence.

At that time only three vitamins had been postulated – to account for the 'deficiency diseases' of scurvy, pellagra and beri-beri. It would be many years before these unknown substances were chemically isolated and identified, and still more before the fifty or so nutrients that are essential for life would be spelled out. Yet the disaster of over-refining of which Dr Williams wrote was by no means the first shift in our evolution to affect our present nutrition.

Since the beginnings of mankind – from *Homo erectus* about one million years ago to *Homo sapiens sapiens* 50,000 years ago – man has been a hunter-gatherer, living partly on the flesh of hunted game, and partly on seeds, nuts and berries gathered from his environment. Archaeologists have shown that we had, long before that time, abandoned living entirely on fruit and leaves. We adapted socially to the use of fire in cooking, to language, to living in small groups of about twenty-five people. The chemist Linus Pauling speculates that the survivors in this nomadic existence were those who were able to move away from the fruit trees of the forests to other sources of ascorbic acid in plant life; thus we evolved into a race that did not need to provide our own vitamin C internally, and then into one that just could not make it ourselves. This loss of use is a strong argument for vitamin supplementation today. In any case, our original diet was clearly a mixed one, not purely vegetarian – even though the length of our intestine, 32 feet as compared with the 12 feet of a meat-eating lion, argues for an emphasis on gathered rather than hunted foods.

Anthropologists point out that our ancestors enjoyed a relatively easy existence in this era, learning to collaborate in the hunting of large animals and, like the present-day hunter-gatherers of southern Africa, the Kung, working only three days a week to maintain an adequate supply of food (the 360 mongongo nuts which a Kung eats a day, for example, provide the protein equivalent of a pound of steak). It appears that our ancestors experimented with mushrooms and other plants for their mind-altering effects, and that fruits were fermented as both preservatives and sedatives.

The first great change in human diet occurred about 10,000 years ago, with the introduction of agriculture. Though there were perhaps only 10 million people on the earth, the Fertile Crescent in the Middle East (the area between the rivers Tigris and Euphrates in present-day Iraq) apparently attracted a sufficiently large population to make farming convenient as well as necessary. It was the start of an astonishing revolution that has significantly distorted our original diet. Mankind now became a consumer – of slave or paid labour, of exotic foods, of all the paraphernalia of settlements. For better or worse, this was the beginning of that social split that exists today in every nation and from nation to nation: the haves and the have nots. From this time we seem to have lost part of the protective mechanism in our bodily constitution that tells us when we have had enough and when we have indulged in what is patently bad for us. Again, it is the story of a human mind capable of rationalising and adjusting for sins of excess as well as for triumphs of creativity.

For all of our recorded history, as if this is how we were from the beginning, we have elevated food to a high level of importance. It is a mother's expression of love, a symbol in courtship, the essential of every religious ritual. A Hindu will not eat cattle, a Jew has strict laws concerning kosher food, and a Moslem will eat only halal. In the Christian tradition, breaking bread is the basic symbol of observance, and every religion has its feasts and its fasts. If a Martian were to land in a modern city he might surmise that our expense-account restaurants are our temples, since this is where we seem to spend so much time.

There is no question that mankind's ability to adapt has mollified the immediate physical effects of the agricultural revolution. The French scientist, René Dubos, writing in the second half of the twentieth century, has called attention to the enormous variation in eating habits around the world; just as we are the tool-makers who can devise a habitat almost anywhere, so our digestive processes seem able to cope with the foods available in the severest conditions. The Masai of Africa live on grains and the produce of cattle; the Eskimos thrive on seals, fish, wild animals, roots and berries. The first is a high-fibre diet, the second a high-fat one. Their incidence of disease is similar. Similarly, the Tibetans live mainly on tea, barley and rancid yak butter – a combination which a nutritionist would deplore for the carcinogenic properties of rancid fats alone. Yet, although they suffer from other medical problems, they are relatively free from the chronic diseases of the industrialised societies.

When we come to the second great revolution in our diet, the introduction of highly processed foods at the end of the nineteenth century and intensifying to our day, it is seductive to think that the debasement of our food supply is alone responsible for the rise in the chronic diseases. The pros and cons of this point have been argued by able researchers on both sides. It is clear that heart disease, which along with stroke accounts for more deaths in our modern society than all the rest of our maladies combined, is related to diet and is not, as some have maintained, simply a disease that previous generations never lived long enough to experience. Atherosclerosis has been observed in autopsies of young soldiers in every war since 1914–18; with each war the levels increase. Yet it is not so clear that sugar alone, or insufficient fibre alone, or a high proportion of fat alone, is the key to this second dietary revolution.

Consider the epidemiologist's assertion that Japanese or Irish or Israelis, when leaving their homeland to live in the United States, soon adopt a similar pattern of chronic disease to that of native Americans. Does it necessarily mean that heart disease increases in the Japanese because of a dietary change, or cancer in the Irish Americans because of processed foods? The danger in such broad comparisons is that it is difficult to take account of all possible changes. It has been suggested that cultural changes, rather than dietary ones, may be primarily responsible for the increased incidence of heart disease in Japanese immigrants to the United States.

With those caveats, therefore, we can now look at the ways in which our eating habits are killing us and consider how we can change them to heal us. Both the farming of our foods, as a result of the modern agricultural revolution, and the processing of our foods, as a result of the marketing revolution, have indeed created problems that our evolutionary mechanisms have not been able to deal with effectively. We know how long it takes to make evolutionary adjustments. For example, many Chinese and Africans find it especially difficult to digest milk products. This is quite different from acquired digestive traits, such as allergies to wheat or shellfish. It may be centuries before entire races may be able to eat the foods that we do; why should it be surprising, then, that we have not been able to adapt to a nutrient-poor food supply, high in fats and low in fibre?

For one reason or another, or a combination of many, the taste buds of the entire human race, and not just Westerners, have become conditioned to the desirability of 'white food': refined sugar, white flour, with the husk extracted, the product of mills invented toward the end of the century, and processed foods of all kinds. In the 1920s, for example, the merchants of Shanghai began to polish the husks off rice to make it look whiter and therefore more attractive to the consumer, not realising that the essential nutrients were in the husks. Diseases such as beri-beri, which in 1890 had been shown by Christiaan Eijkman to be the result of a deficiency in polished rice, promptly appeared, and were not conquered until the polishing process was made less efficient. It was a sign of wealth in many countries to avoid the black bread of peasants; and the desired whiteness was sometimes achieved by the use of lead, which had also been used for centuries in cosmetics. We now know that lead poisoning is among the most insidious of the environmental hazards of our industrial society. We are attempting to remove it from most petrol; it is banned in children's toys, domestic piping and paint. High concentrations of lead have been correlated with high prison populations in Switzerland and elsewhere. Learning disabilities have been shown to rise with serum lead levels. It has been speculated that an entire civilisation was undermined by the use of lead glaze in cooking pots and as a wine sweetener: the Roman Empire.

The food industry acknowledges all the dangers of environmental poisons, and indeed continually jousts with government agencies over the merits of this or that sweetener, this or that preservative. The industry's spokesmen contend that food processing, which now accounts for more than 60 per cent of the value of all food consumed in industrialised countries, is a necessary adjunct of such a society. Our large urban populations could not obtain even the basic foodstuffs, not to mention canned and frozen foods from other countries, without extensive processing. It is better for children to be inveigled into eating a breakfast of sugared flakes than for them not to eat anything at all. The cost of living would rise precipitously if everyone had to shop for all their vegetables in fresh form. Besides, people today don't have the time or the inclination to spend hours over food preparation. Food manufacturers, in short, are simply doing for us what we want – or so the argument goes.

This point of view would not be remarkable except for the tacit support of the food industry by organised medicine and the media, who are dependent on their supply of recommendations and data. Many crusaders have campaigned for a return to wholesome foods – though they are often characterised as quacks by the medical and food establishment – but none has been so powerful as public opinion. The popularisers all had their adherents, going back to Bernard MacFadden and Carlton Fredericks, Adele Davis and, from the highest scientific ranks, Roger Williams and Linus Pauling. Yet the popularisers constituted a threat to medical schools, hospital dieticians, medical associations and industry journals. It was the general public, and not the scientific community, that kept nutrition alive as a viable alternative to drug therapy. The most striking evidence of this today is the popularity of the healthfood shop, even with its array of dubious products and reliance on fad diets. The issue comes down clearly to the role of vitamins and minerals as supplements. Is our food supply so bad that such supplements are needed?

The standard answer of virtually every medical text, and most of the newspaper columnists who rely on the food industry and the medical associations for information, is that a 'balanced diet' is adequate for all our nutritional needs and is, in addition, available to anyone with commonsense and even a minimal income. This answer flouts decades of research, going back to studies of poor populations of London in the 1930s, and continuing into the 1980s. It, in fact, requires knowledge and dedication to achieve a balanced food intake, and even then it may not provide what we really need. In the United States, the Health and Nutrition Examination Surveys have consistently exposed widespread deficiencies in this supposedly affluent society. In a sample made in 1971–4, half of all adult men between twenty-five and fifty-four, and women between twenty and forty-four, were below the recommended daily allowance (RDA) for vitamin C. In 1982, half of all women in the USA over the age of fifteen were deficient in protein – and this supposedly a protein-conscious society. These are some of the obvious deficiencies; women have been reported seriously deficient in iron for decades in the United States; deficiencies occur throughout the minerals; and for the trace minerals sufficient standards do not exist yet that would enable any reliable evaluation to be made. The answer of consumerists and nutritionists to the 'balanced diet' theory is simply that there is no evidence that there has been any such animal throughout this century.

The disputed case of vitamin C is a good example of the intricacies of the 'food as healer' issue. When, during the 1960s, it was brought to the front pages of the daily newspapers by Linus Pauling's startling presentation of ascorbic acid as the answer to the common cold, a 'megadose' controversy erupted. Pauling recommended as much as 8 grams of vitamin C a day, arguing that this amount is in the range of what an animal produces relative to its weight. In the case of an onset of a cold, he suggested a gram or more an hour. The Food and Nutrition Board of the National Academy of Sciences in the United States considered less than 50 milligrams sufficient per day – the RDA. Pauling's intake was 200 times that amount!

In spite of claims of possible side effects on kidney stones, Pauling would admit no dangers in these megadoses beyond what he termed 'bowel tolerance'. If one experienced diarrhoea, it would quickly subside by stopping the vitamin C intake: this was a sign of a healthy metabolism. If, on the other hand, increasing doses induced no bowel problems, the ascorbic acid could be considered to be working against disease. Many doctors began treating heavy respiratory illnesses with 50–60 grams a day. Meanwhile, the scientific community conducted a few double-blind studies – a placebo versus a gram of vitamin C; they were inconclusive. Pauling has since been castigated for his claims for vitamin C treatment – he also considered that it was effective in treating cancer. Few people remember that penicillin, too, was not effective when it was originally tested on some diseases – because it was given in too small a dose. The idea of treating a cold with one gram of vitamin C a day is like taking just a little penicillin.

Pauling's recommendation for taking 200 times the RDA, or the average health nut's habit of 2–3 grams – forty or sixty times the RDA – brings up the question of how RDAs were established. The answer is simple: enough of each nutrient was recommended to prevent the deficiency diseases, with a margin of error thrown in to compensate for 'individual differences'. As the American scientist, Roger Williams, has shown, biochemical differences can vary by factors of 20 or 30 from one individual to another; at best we can say that the RDA is a move in the right direction. The amount of ascorbate needed to prevent scurvy was established in the 1930s, by Dr William Hodges, at about 10 milligrams. This was the figure used by the Food and Nutrition Board in 1943 to set its first RDA for vitamin C. Richard Hawkins had used citrus juice in 1593 to alleviate scurvy among English sailors. A century and a half later, the Scottish physician James Lind conducted what we would call controlled experiments of a concentrated form of orange juice – the first megavitamin! – extending the voyages of British ships for three months. It took an additional two centuries for this mysterious 'anti-scurvy' factor, or ascorbate, to be isolated in the lab.

In the parade of discoveries since that time – the B vitamins, not completed until 1973; the trace minerals, several of which were found after 1974 to have a biological role – the general public has been victimised by another, parallel development in medical science: drugs. We have seen how the idea of 'magic bullets', capable of acting on specific parts of the body, was considered preposterous before Ehrlich's discovery of 606, as described in Chapter 5. Yet throughout the twenties, thirties and forties, when antibiotics were being developed as just these magic bullets, vitamins and minerals were being synthesised or isolated. It was inescapable that these also would be considered single-purpose agents. Wasn't ascorbate the answer to scurvy? Wasn't beri-beri cured by B vitamins, and pellagra by niacin?

As a result, charts and graphs were designed to tell us what vitamin or trace element to take for each ailment: for stress, B vitamins; for sexual potency, zinc (hence the claims for oysters); for building the heart, vitamin E; for night blindness, vitamin A; for a better memory, choline; for blood-clotting, vitamin K. To wander into a healthfood shop is to be in the presence of an alchemist; the vitamin and mineral 'industry' is trying to mimic the pharmaceutical companies.

It will take time, but eventually people will learn that supplements are probably useless as magic bullets. Each nutrient needs others to be metabolised; all work in a synergistic way. This does not mean that vitamin C in megadoses won't work: it will work better if the B complex and E are also present. Zinc may be washed out of our systems if they lack magnesium for absorption. This is why a balanced diet, if it could be achieved, is indeed best for us. So far man has uncovered about fifty nutrients: some thirteen vitamins, ten essential amino acids, three essential fatty acids, six major minerals and fifteen trace elements. All of these are needed to turn glucose into energy which we can use.

If you think you have no need for vitamin supplements, take note of the research by Dr Hughes at the University of Wales. He fed the diet of a Welsh farm labourer and a typical modern diet to mice. On the modern diet, the laboratory animals died relatively young.

A growing concern of our day, if not as pressing as that of nuclear annihilation, is the violence in our society that is exemplified both by aggressiveness in the young and by rising lawlessness in general. There have been many studies aimed at the food–behaviour connection. The Scots used to explain their morning porridge with the aphoristic 'It sticks to your ribs'; yet it is simply the slow digestion of oats, or other fibrous foods, that supplies a regular flow of energy – in contrast to the rush of insulin following a high-sugar breakfast, which in turn causes abnormally low blood sugar and consequent food cravings. This so-called hypoglycaemic reaction has been blamed for many of the emotional ills of young people on a typical processed food diet. Large numbers of seemingly innocent foods, such as tomato ketchup, conceal excessive amounts of sugar. The soft drinks and breakfast food markets are obvious examples. Problems in schools, either from poor performance or from bad behaviour, have spread throughout society in an ominous correlation with the rise in the consumption of sugar and junk food.

The work of a young scientist called Alexander Schauss is typical of the innovative research being done today against the background of behavioural problems, as defined by one of his prominent papers,

'Diet, Crime and Delinquency'. Dr Schauss' approach is typical of the cautious, practical investigative work that is going on at the present time in Britain and America. His story is crucial to the case for nutrition as a social corrective.

Coming to the United States from Germany as a child in 1955, Schauss went on to study music and social science before becoming a probation officer – the youngest ever appointed in the USA. He had been intrigued by summer work in New York City with heroin addicts, noting that some were the only member of their family to behave in this way. In one of his first cases he received a shock that was to set him on the course of his life's work. A young boy with an extensive criminal record was placed in his charge, and Schauss had to recommend the court to send him to reform school for four years. A vigorous defence counsel demanded a physiological examination, and an expert in genetics was called in. It was quickly determined that the boy had no secondary sex characteristics, had been concealing this disability, and accordingly had exhibited anti-social behaviour because of conflicts with his demanding 'macho' father. The boy was successfully treated with nutrition and physiotherapy – but the lesson for Dr Schauss was that grave injustices were easy to commit because the causes of anti-social behaviour were seldom sought. In the courts in which he had worked, this was the first physiological referral in twenty-one years.

Four years later, as the youngest planner appointed to the US Institute of Justice, Dr Schauss pursued the connection between nutrition and behaviour. He noticed that the average length of stay in reformatories was eighteen months, yet in one case it was only four months. Why was this one different? On careful examination he found that the only anomaly was that this institution either grew its own food or purchased it from local farmers – and did not use sugar or additives in its preparation. A few years later, Dr Schauss was in a position to organise a controlled experiment to test this intriguing hypothesis. Now a probation officer working with adults, he set up three groups of adult offenders: the first was left on their normal diet; the second was instructed in good eating habits; the third was also taught how to cook. The normal re-arrest rate of 35 per cent occurred in the first group, but this dropped to 18 and 11 per cent respectively in the other two.

When this result was reported in the paper mentioned above, the distinguished criminologist Dr Stephen Schonfield rebutted that in the huge literature of criminal behaviour a link with diet had never been suggested. Schauss replied that if genetics could be considered a factor, why not eating – an action that affects us daily. Schonfield decided to conduct his own dietary experiments; to his surprise, they confirmed Schauss' work. However, this type of nutritional research continues to cause argument amongst scientists.

Dr Schauss is now the director of an organisation that continues such studies – the American Institute for Bio-Social Studies in Tacoma, Washington. In research on delinquent and normal children in matched groups, he was unable to make any correlations between food additives or sugar and errant behaviour. Yet he did uncover unusual patterns of nutrition. In one group, some delinquents were drinking 15–20 pints of milk a day. This excellent food was hardly the cause of delinquency, but it did reveal a severe imbalance in eating habits. When added to such habits as smoking, heavy coffee drinking and large consumption of phosphates in soft drinks, this unusual calorific intake undoubtedly resulted in a distorted absorption of minerals and vitamins.

In other controversial studies with delinquents and control groups in a town near Washington DC – a very prosperous community where malnutrition is unlikely – the substitution of orange juice or water for milk resulted in a decrease in anti-social behaviour by 47 per cent. Clearly, vitamin C in the orange juice alone was not responsible for the change. The complex interactions of nutrients are impossible to predict in broad epidemiological studies; but it is known that vitamin C assists in the uptake of iron from sources other than meat, and that low levels of iron are correlated with low academic achievement. In severe anaemia, the cognitive processes of the left side of the brain are hampered. In addition orange juice contains thiamin and folic acid, also necessary for full use of the brain.

Dr Schauss' work has involved him in large-scale prison studies concerning the effects on behaviour not only of nutrition, but also of exercise, full-spectrum lighting and colour. One notable study concerns the correlation of the chronic diseases in Western society with the concomitant decline in examination marks and the rise in delinquency in schools in the United States. Published as *The Ford Report on the Impact of Nutrition on the Health of Americans*, this study has now been expanded into areas of environment, life-style and genetics. It has been acutely observed that we do not lack for studies, but we do lack a nation or even a community able to translate the research into action.

At present numerous medical and para-medical societies exist, in

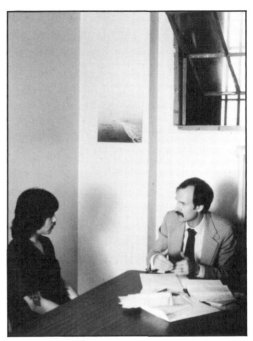

Alex Schauss interviewing a young prisoner in Lewis County Jail, Washington. He is investigating the possibility of a link between the prisoner's alcoholism and drug-taking and his long-term dietary deficiencies

the United States and Britain, with the aim of promoting the nutritional component of health care. Techniques of analysis have been carefully worked out: computerised dietary analyses, vitamin and mineral assays, glucose tolerance tests and even amino acid assays. Diagnostic procedures have become standardised through exchanges in medical journals. Contaminants in foods and in the environment can now be easily tested, as can allergic reactions. Yet a significant problem remains in that the medical doctors who specialise in this form of treatment are fragmented by their inability to communicate through the orthodox medical profession.

We should remind ourselves that progress is often measured in centuries – as in the case of James Lind and scurvy. That common nutritional problem – being overweight – is still treated by most practitioners as a 'calories in, calories out' proposition. But the body is neither a machine nor a test tube; its internal mechanisms still confound us. Writing in 1921, in the article referred to at the beginning of this chapter, Dr Leonard Williams expressed the hope that 'the ineffable theory of calories which is based on the curious assumption that the behaviour of food in the human body was identical with is behaviour in the test tube, will retire to the limbo of things well forgotten'.

EPILOGUE

A journey is not a round tour; it does not return home, and it does not even necessarily end. A journey is an invitation to discovery, not a catalogue of discoveries. We hope that in retelling our experiences we have brought you to your own discoveries rather than to ours.

We first asked how to determine when a person was ill. It was suggested in the Bible: 'The heart knoweth its own bitterness.'

We looked at the scientific medicine of the West from Eastern eyes, and found that it has *yang*. It questions itself. In its aggressiveness it makes many errors, but it has a mechanism to right itself, and then to go deeper into the quest for truth. It is sanguine in its self-confidence, and it sometimes forgets that it is balanced by the shady side of the slope, by *yin*.

We admired the ancient arts of medicine because they are ancient as well as current to our needs. Yet their survival is not what gives them a claim to credence. When they do confirm what we now experience to be true, they speak to us on the continuity of the human spirit.

We told stories about the great healers of the past, some of them considered charlatans, to try to bring to life the drama that exists in our daily struggle for existence. We tried to use these key figures to divide the history of medicine into comprehensible parts, and to show why we have the medicine we do in the twentieth century.

We would like to leave a vision of medicine that includes all human striving for wellness. We see illness not as an aberration, but as an essential part of being alive. Music would not be possible without the suspension of finality, without minor chords striving for resolution. Life, like music, is inherently unresolved. But from time to time we are blessed with finales, and we realise that a finale is no more the whole of music than health is the whole of life. The healing arts will always be part of our lives.

FURTHER·READING

The literature concerning medicine and health is obviously vast. The following introductory books are our suggestions for anyone wanting to pursue more deeply the issues we have raised during this journey through the healing arts.

1 The Balanced Way
FILLIOZAT, J. *The classical doctrine of Indian medicine* Delhi: Munshiram Manoharlal, 1964.
HUARD, P. and WONG, M. *Chinese medicine* New York: McGraw-Hill, 1968.
JAGGI, O. P. *Indian system of medicine* Delhi: Atma Ram, 1973.
KAPTCHUK, T. J. *Chinese medicine: the web that has no weaver* London: Rider, 1983.
LESLIE, C. *Asian medical systems* Berkeley: University of California Press, n.e. 1976.
MAJNO, G. *The healing hand: man and wound in the ancient world* Cambridge, Massachusetts: Harvard University Press, 1975.
PHILLIPS, E. D. *Aspects of Greek medicine* New York: St Martin's Press, 1973.
TEMKIN, O. *Galenism: rise and decline of a medical philosophy* Ithaca, New York: Cornell University Press, 1973. op.

2 The Mystery of Illness
COCHRANE, A. L. *Effectiveness and efficiency: random reflections on the health services* London: Nuffield Provincial Hospital Trust, Oxford University Press, 1972. op.
FABREGA, H. *Disease and social behavior* Cambridge, Massachusetts: MIT Press, 1974.
HELMAN, C. *Culture, health and illness* Bristol: Wright, 1984.
KLEINMAN, A. *Patients and healers in the context of culture* Berkeley: University of California Press, n.e. 1981.
McKEOWN, T. *The role of medicine* Princeton: Princeton University Press, 1979.
WRIGHT, P. and ANDREW, T. *The problem of medical knowledge* Edinburgh: Edinburgh University Press, 1982.
ZOLA, I. K. *Socio-medical inquiries* Philadelphia: Temple University Press, 1983.

3 Hands On
BISHOP, W. J. *The early history of surgery* Robert Hale, 1960. op.

165

COWIE, J. B. and ROEBUCK, J. B. *An ethnography of a chiropractic clinic* New York: Free Press, 1975.
GEVITZ, N. *The D.O.'s: osteopathic medicine in America* Baltimore: Johns Hopkins University Press, 1982.
MONTAGU, A. *Touching: the human significance of the skin* New York: Harper and Row, n.e. 1979.
SCHIOTZ, E. H. and CYRIAX, J. *Manipulation, past and present* London: William Heinemann Medical Books, 1975.

4 Nature's Green Pharmacy
ACKERKNECHT, E. H. *Therapeutics: from the primitive to the 20th century* New York: Hafner Press, 1973.
GRIGGS, B. *Green pharmacy: a history of herbal medicine* London: Norman and Hobhouse, 1982.
INGLIS, B. *History of medicine* London: Weidenfeld and Nicolson, 1965.
SIGERIST, H. E. *A history of medicine* New York: Oxford University Press, 1977.
WHEELWRIGHT, E. G. *Medicinal plants and their history* New York: Dover, 1974.

5 Enter Magic Bullets
COULTER, H. L. *Divided legacy: a history of the schism in medical thought* 3 vols. Washington, D.C.: Wehawken Book Co., 1973–5.
DEKRUIF, P. *Microbe hunters* New York: Harcourt, Brace and Co., 1926.
MELVILLE, A. *Cured to death: the effects of prescription drugs* New York: Stein and Day, 1982.
PAGEL, W. *Paracelsus* New York: S. Karger, 2nd edn. 1982.
VITHOULKAS, G. *The science of homeopathy* New York: Grove Press, 1982.
WEINER, M. and GOSS, K. *The complete book of homeopathy* New York: Bantam Books, 1982.

6 The Mind Wants Back In
ALEXANDER, F. *Psychosomatic medicine* New York: W. W. Norton, 1965.
BENSON, H. and PROCTOR, W. *Beyond the relaxation response* New York: Times Books, 1984.
ELLENBERGER, H. F. *The discovery of the unconscious* New York: Basic Books, 1970.
ENTRALGO, P. L. *Mind and body* London: Harvill, 1955.
FRANK, J. D. *Persuasion and healing* Baltimore: Johns Hopkins Press, 1961. op; Schocken, rev. edn. 1974.
PELLETIER, K. R. *Mind as healer, mind as slayer* New York: Delacorte, 1977.
SELYE, H. *The stress of life* New York: McGraw-Hill, n.e. 1978.

7 The Return of Ritual
BERMAN, M. *The reenchantment of the world* New York: Bantam Books, 1984.
ELIADE, M. *Shamanism* Princeton, New Jersey: Princeton University Press, 1974.
EVANS-PRITCHARD, E. E. *Witchcraft, oracles and magic among the Azande* OUP, 1976.
KIEV, A., ed. *Magic, faith and healing* Macmillan, 1974. op.

MIDDLETON, J., ed. *Magic, witchcraft, and curing* University of Texas, 1976.

ROGERS, S. L. *The shaman* Springfield, Illinois: Charles C. Thomas, 1982.

TILLICH, P. *The meaning of health* Richmond, California: North Atlantic Books, 1981.

8 The Open Clinic

BAKAN, D. *Disease, pain and sacrifice* Boston: Beacon Press, 1971.

CASSELL, E. J. *The healer's art* New York: Penguin Books, 1978. op.

LEVINE, S. *Who dies?* Garden City, New York: Anchor Books, 1982.

MELZACK, R. and WALL, P. D. *The challenge of pain* New York: Basic Books, 1983.

WEIL, A. *Health and healing* Boston: Houghton Mifflin, 1983.

9 & 10 The Lost Art of Moving and Eating

CANNON, C. *Dieting makes you fat* London: Century, 1983.

DAVIES, S. and STEWART, A. *Nutritional medicine* London: Pan, 1986.

EISENBERG, D. *Encounters with qi: exploring Chinese medicine* New York: W. W. Norton, 1985; London: Jonathan Cape, 1986.

FELDENKRAIS, M. *Body and mature behavior* New York: International Universities, 1979.

GRIGGS, B. *The food factor* London: Viking, 1986.

REID, H. and CROUCHER, M. *The way of the warrior* London: Century, 1983.

PICTURE · CREDITS

INDEX

Page numbers in *italic* refer to the illustrations and captions